Taking My Medicine

My Journey from Teenage Mother to Physician

* * *

Melanie Watkins, M.D.

This is a non-fiction story. It is based my life experiences as a teenager and young adult. For this memoir, I referred frequently to journals that I have kept since my adolescence. Throughout this book, I have tried to maintain my 'voice'—meaning the reactions that I had about people, places, topics and ideas were genuinely how I felt during my adolescence and young adulthood at the times I was experiencing them. Now, as an adult, I do not necessarily have the same perspective or opinions, but I have tried to keep the writing true to my thoughts and feelings as a young person. Occasionally, some names and identifying characteristics have been changed to protect privacy.

* * *

Dedication

To Jonathan: your name means "Gift from God". You have been such a blessing to me and I am proud to be your mother. May you be successful in the way that you define success.

To pregnant and parenting teenagers: life can be challenging trying to figure out who you are and your place in this world while raising children. May you always know you have a voice and a choice. May you have the courage to live the life each of you is capable of living.

* * *

Listening to my baby's heartbeat

Is like listening to the horses galloping in the fields

Running free

I wish we could be free

Be free like runaway horses

That never, ever look back

--Melanie Watkins, age sixteen

Introduction

My grandfather died in the summer of 1989. That was the first time the right side of my head throbbed so badly that I became nauseated. Lights were too bright, sound was too loud, and no one in my family had a name for this killer pain—migraines. I'd lie in bed, curled in a fetal position, not knowing what was happening to me.

I was thirteen at the time, and I'd spent many summers at my grandparents' home near Shreveport. Their house was a bit run-down—not unusual for a farm in northwest Louisiana—but the rooster greeted the dawn each morning, and my grandmother prepared wonderful meals in the kitchen morning, noon, and night. After all these years, I can still smell that house—the simple furniture, the bedding, the floorboards, the curtains. The house had been lived in by good people, and I instinctively knew that it was a good place to be—a *safe* place to be.

Like most kids, I was observant, looking for the rhythms of life. I watched my grandmother remove insulin vials from the refrigerator so that my grandfather, a diabetic, could receive his shots. My grandmother folded laundry and did chores while farm animals wandered around the yard. The screen door banged against the jamb as people came and went. On Sundays we went to church and sang hymns. I was welcome there, part of a daily routine, part of a family.

The best part of these summer visits was listening to my grandfather tell stories. Whether they were Biblical in nature or traditional fables, they always had a point, a moral that my grandfather wished to impart. In fact, my grandparents were both deeply religious, and my grandmother always made sure I didn't roll up my jeans too high or wear make-up—made sure, as the Bible says, that I did not conform to the things of this world. At night, grandma would kneel with me next to my bed and make sure I said my prayers. It was on these nights that I learned how to talk to God.

After enjoying such wonderful summers in the past, coping with my grandfather's death in 1989 was difficult. My mother put me on Greyhound bus and sent me to Louisiana so that I could help out in whatever way I could. I tried to give my grandmother support by cooking lunch and dinner and looking after my six-year-old cousin, T. J. I cooked and cleaned more than I ever had in my entire life. It was a heavy burden for someone so young, and the house now smelled like sadness more than anything else.

The migraine hit, and my grandmother had me lie down on her bed. I held my head in my hands, and if someone could have removed the right side of my brain, I would have offered no resistance. The headache was made worse because guilt and fear mingled with the actual pain. How could I cook dinner? How could I sweep and dust and mop and take care of my cousin? I needed to take care of grandma, but now she was taking care of me. I had become a burden, not an asset, but the pain was so bad that I wondered if I might be dying. That's not a topic that a thirteen year old should have to consider.

My grandmother didn't know what was wrong with me—this obviously wasn't an ordinary headache—but she prayed for me and asked someone from her local church to come by and anoint my head with oil, and the headache finally began to slide away. The guilt dissipated as I relaxed in grandma's arms, allowing myself to be cared for. It was as if a dozen small streams were draining from a lake of pain that had formed inside my head. The throbbing was gone.

There would be other migraines, however, and a great deal more stress in my life—more than I could possibly imagine. The peaceful days of feeling connected to a family—of feeling wanted—were destined to disappear. The horrible lake of pain would fill up many more times.

* * *

1

My mother and I moved from Phoenix to Jackson, Mississippi in 1991, when I was fifteen. My mother was a government employee, and at age forty-five, she'd taken a job in Jackson with the Corps of Engineers since her U.S. government pay grade was higher there. Within a week of our arrival, my mother, Dorothy Watkins, enrolled me in Callaway High, a school I instantly disliked. In Phoenix, I'd attended Trevor Browne High School—a school with far more cultural and ethnic diversity. It's where my friends were. I didn't fit in at Callaway, where I experienced culture shock of the worst kind. Where were the white students? A few lived in my neighborhood, but for the most part, they attended Murrah High School, which was five miles away. Murrah looked more like a college than a high school, with a modern lobby and classrooms. Even its athletic uniforms were nicer. At Callaway, the classrooms were mostly a maze of modular trailers that bore no resemblance to the ordered halls and classrooms in Phoenix. All special events at my new school had to be funded by the old-fashioned, tedious method of selling candy door-to-door, which most definitely wasn't the case at the more affluent Murrah.

I was isolated, lonely. Kids at Callaway made fun of the way I talked and dressed. I "talked white," as they termed it. I also wore more casual clothing, such as jeans and a T-shirt, which was the norm for the more laid-back lifestyle of the West Coast. Despite Callaway's sharp contrast with Murrah, the students nevertheless placed great emphasis on designer jeans and shoes. I found this difficult to process. It was 1991, not 1961. Why did my speech or clothes matter? Hadn't society gotten beyond such superficialities? Accordingly, I resented my mother for putting me into this time warp, where old divisions and stereotypes still existed.

Fortunately, I had at least one good friend at Callaway. Sandra was in my tenth-grade geometry class, and she invited me to a Bible study at the local Baptist church. Reluctant to give me much freedom in a new environment, my mother begrudgingly agreed to let me attend. I guess she thought I couldn't get in very much trouble at church. She would soon come to regret the decision.

Everyone was warm and welcoming at the church's youth event, accepting me for who I was—a far cry from the atmosphere at Callaway. It had been a long time since my mother and I had been to church, but I had continued to pray thanks to my grandparents' example during those summers in Louisiana. (I had already prayed on more than one occasion to either be accepted in Jackson or be allowed to leave, but God had thus far remained silent.) But on that fall evening in 1991, no one pointed out my differences. I was simply Melanie Watkins, a child of God.

The Bible study finished around 7 p.m., at which time Sandra and I walked under the dark evening sky into the parking lot, where her mother was scheduled to pick us up. While we waited, someone at the end of the parking lot tried to get my attention.

"Hey, girl!" called a male voice.

I turned my head to see who the voice belonged to. Who could possibly know me at this small Baptist church in Jackson "far-from-from-everywhere" Mississippi?

"Yeah, you—you right there. You with the black skirt."

At the end of the lot, a muscular man smoking a cigarette leaned against his sports car, an older green model that had probably had been tweaked for power and volume. He sported jeans, tight T-shirt, and a military-style haircut, silver dog tags dangling around his neck. Tattoos curled around his large, rounded biceps.

"Do you know that guy?" I asked Sandra, giggling.

"No," she answered, smiling. "But he sure is looking hard at you—*real* hard."

"Come over here for a minute," the young man shouted. "Let's talk."

I could tell instantly that he was older than I. I was fifteen, and if he was in the military, he had to be at least eighteen.

"Stay with me, Sandra," I said, nervously approaching him.

Sandra stood close by for support as I reached his car.

"What's your name, girl?" asked the young man.

"Melanie," I said softly.

He grinned. "Melllahhhneeeeee," he said, emphasizing every syllable with his southern accent. He shook his head back and forth, staring me up and down. "Melanie, Melanie, Melanie," he repeated.

It was a scene from a movie, the young innocent girl slowly succumbing to the flirtations of an older man.

I turned away and smiled nervously at Sandra, my heart racing. The muscular man who had taken a sudden interest in me was both intriguing and intimidating.

"Can I call you sometime, Melanie?" he asked nonchalantly, blowing a column of smoke into the night air.

"My mom doesn't allow me to get calls from boys," I replied.

He seemed unfazed, flicking his cigarette to the side and stepping on it. "I'm a man. You call me. Your mom ain't got to know about me." His tone was insistent. He wrote his number on a piece of scrap paper—Darryl, 555-5678—and handed it to me.

Still behind me, Sandra leaned close and whispered in my ear. "Melanie, we gotta go. My mom is gonna kill us if she sees us over here."

She was right, of course, but I was drawn to Darryl's self-confidence.

"I have to go, Darryl," I said, trying to control my giddiness.

"Call me," he reiterated, flashing a wide grin as he crossed his arms.

I smiled at him and walked away just in time to see Sandra's mother pulling into the parking lot.

I was still alone in Jackson, but not as alone as before. There was Sandra, as well as the kids in the church youth group.

And there was Darryl.

* * *

2

My courtship with Darryl began within days. He would pick me up from school, buy me a fast food snack, and drop me off just before my mom got home from work. It was pretty straightforward at first—a ride home, a snack, a little conversation—but it didn't stay that way.

Over the next six months, Darryl, who was twenty years old and in the Army Reserves, checked me out of school on days I didn't skip out altogether. I didn't have much motivation to apply myself academically since the faculty and staff didn't challenge their students. Test scores at the school were low, and my normal study habits—nose to the grindstone all the way—soon dissolved. I had tried to belong, joining the French Club, the Future Business Leaders of America, and the cheerleading squad, but the other kids continued to tease me about my speech and clothing. I even ran for student council—I was more than qualified—but I wasn't one of the beautiful, popular kids. Callaway, therefore, had no redeeming features. School was boring. That my mom had uprooted me from the life and schools I'd enjoyed in Phoenix was always at the forefront of my mind. Consequently, any guilt I experienced for ditching school rapidly dissipated.

More than anything, however, Darryl's magnetic pull helped me overcome any fear that I might get caught. Other than Sandra and her Baptist youth group, he was the only good thing I'd discovered in Jackson. He accepted and loved everything about me—mannerisms, dress, accent—everything that the other kids disdained. Ironically, having an older boyfriend actually provided me with a bit of status among my peers, not that it won me any close friends.

My resentment for my mother grew exponentially with each passing day. Darryl had a bit of a bad boy mentality, and I knew that my mother would thoroughly disapprove of him. But that was okay by me. I was finishing my sophomore year at a high school where I didn't belong. What my mother thought was irrelevant.

* * *

Darryl never apologized for who he was, and he told me to do the same—to never be ashamed of who I was or what I felt. This advice resonated with a Phoenix transplant in the midst of lethargic, intolerant Jackson. I enjoyed his company, mostly because he seemed to genuinely care about me. He bought me flowers and candy, and during the days when I was eluding the humdrum classes at Callaway, Darryl and I went to the park, the movies, or just hung out. Sometimes we were intimate. He was a man who was confident and in complete control.

Sometimes, however, control has a dark side. He always wanted to know the schedules for my classes or cheerleading practice. He insisted on knowing who I was with at any given time—and why. I merely attributed his concern for my whereabouts to the broader fact that he cared about me as a person. When things didn't go his way, however—if his well laid plans or itinerary for our activities were disrupted—he began manifesting a temper that was downright scary. He made it abundantly clear that I was not to spend time with friends and that any time away from home or school was to be spent with him. I started walking on eggshells, choosing my words and actions carefully. These demands were totally unreasonable, of course, but I dared not awaken his anger if at all possible. His anger was a light sleeper.

Still, I wasn't willing to give Darryl up, even though I found this aspect of his personality more than a bit disquieting. He was all I had, and if my being with him upset my mother, so much the better. Being Darryl's girlfriend was worth the risk.

* * *

Ironically, Mom was also having a hard time adjusting to life in Jackson, but at least she had a good-paying job. She wasn't especially connected to the city, but her work provided her with routine and focus. I had neither, only my twenty-year-old boyfriend. I eventually gave my number to Darryl just to see if he could get away with calling my home at a predetermined time without my mother knowing about the clandestine communication. It was part of my defiance, but it didn't work. Mom found out in short order, and when Darryl called, she would say, "Don't call my daughter anymore!" before hanging up.

Because of calls from Callaway's main office, Mom also learned that I had been skipping school. Needless to say, this disclosure only increased our alienation from one another. I began talking back to mom, expressing "attitude" that comes easily to a fifteen year old. While mom had always taken care of the necessities of life—food, clothing, shelter—she was distant rather than nurturing. Now, in Jackson, she seemed more than just distant. She was strict and mean, appearing oblivious to the fact that my very rewarding life in Phoenix, from kindergarten through high school, had been summarily taken away. I didn't begrudge her making more money at a new job, but what about my own needs? Didn't they count as well?

I soon found out that Mom and my sister Tonya had been discussing my situation over the phone. In most homes, the buck gets passed with the traditional "Talk with your father" when a child isn't behaving. My father, Melvin, had dropped out of my life when I was very young. He occasionally showed up for special events, like a birthday or spelling bee, but he was basically AWOL, so requesting my dad to rein me in wasn't an option. That task fell to Tonya, who was ten years older than I.

Tonya had not gotten along well with Mom either. She'd felt so controlled by Dot, as she called my mother, that she moved out of our home in Phoenix on her eighteenth birthday. That was now water under the bridge, but Mom feared that I might also leave home or, worse yet, that Darryl might take me away. When my mother got exasperated with my behavior, therefore, I was told to call Tonya. She thought I might be more open to the words of a sibling.

Unfortunately, Tonya was dealing with her own struggles. At twenty-five, she was separated from her husband and raising her daughter Sloane under difficult financial circumstances. We were both enduring severe hardships, but that didn't stop Tonya from trying to calm the troubled domestic waters in Jackson with a little bit of tough love. Basically, she was Mom's surrogate.

"Hey, little sister," Tonya told me one night on the phone. "What's going on over there? Dot says you've been acting up."

Tonya always got straight to the point. Long distance was expensive, and there was no time for small talk.

"I don't really know what's going on," I answered, "except that Mom is mean. She doesn't like my boyfriend and won't let me do anything! I hate it here. Life was much better in Phoenix."

Tonya sighed. "You're living under Mom's roof, so you need to live by her rules. I know she's difficult, but you need to focus on school and do what you have to do."

Easier said than done, I thought.

"Tonya, can I come live with you?" I blurted the words out in desperation, as if my tongue had a mind of its own. "Please! I'll get a job and help out with Sloane. I won't bother you—I promise—but I can't take it here anymore."

"Melanie, things here are hard right now. I can barely keep food on the table. Besides, I don't think Dot would allow it."

I started to cry. "I'm going to be a junior this fall. I miss Phoenix, and the worst part is that I'm not learning anything here. Nothing at all. My school doesn't care about anybody."

"Well, you might learn something if you bothered to go to class."

The words stung more than a little. I was being chastised by my own sister, someone who should have been able to empathize with me.

"I'm bored when I go to class," I told her. "I already know everything they're teaching. I want to be a doctor, but at this rate, I won't even be able to get into college."

I was being a bit melodramatic, but that's what the situation called for. Neither Mom nor Tonya had a college degree. They both knew I was smart, so why wouldn't they want me to be the first in our family to attend a university?

Tonya was silent for a few long minutes.

"Okay," she said. "I'll talk with Dot and see what I can do. I'm not sure how to make this work, or if I would even be considered your legal guardian."

"Thank you!" I said excitedly. "Thank you so much!"

My prayers had been answered, after all—maybe. Mom had to sign off on the deal.

I handed the phone to Mom, who talked to Tonya while I paced nervously in the adjoining dining room. That's when thoughts of Darryl swam into my mind. How could I face him? What would I say? His temper would erupt like a volcano if he knew I was planning to leave Jackson, but I knew one thing for certain: I wasn't getting anywhere with Mom and Darryl controlling me all the time. The pressure had become intolerable. Mom was aloof, Darryl's temper was always seething just below the surface, but I had to keep everything bottled up for the most part.

Mom was cooking while she talked with Tonya for half an hour. Her voice sounded disinterested, spent. Was she going to exert her parental control just because that was her privilege, or was she fed up, ready to let me go? When Mom finally emerged into the dining room, I was sitting in a chair, pretending to be engrossed in a magazine.

"You can move back to Phoenix and live with Tonya," she said matter-of-factly. "She'll be your legal guardian. If you want to try to do this on your own, then go right ahead."

There was a definite undertone of "You're going to fail" in her weary voice, but at least she had relented. I was leaving dreary Jackson for Phoenix, the only real home I'd ever known.

And yet I looked hard at my mother as she gave me permission to leave. Didn't she want me? It had almost been too simple. One conversation with Tonya, and I was gone—just like that. My mother informed me that I could leave whenever I wanted. Meanwhile, Tonya would enroll me in school.

I wanted to live with Tonya, but I was conflicted. It would have been nice if Mom had displayed a bit more emotion, maybe even a bit of sadness that I was leaving the nest.

Sadly, that's not who my mother was.

* * *

3

The summer of 1992 was a good time to move. Junior year was just around the corner, and I could rekindle my scholastic ambitions. I was nervous—this was the first time I was leaving home—but excited about once again living in Phoenix. I packed everything I owned in a large suitcase—clothes, mementos, and books, the latter being Stephen King novels, *Seventeen* magazine, and other paperbacks popular among my age group. I closed the case, studied it for a moment, and thought *this is everything that's mine. This is quite literally me—who I am.*

Then it was off to the bus station, where I realized I had to call Darryl. I had no idea whatsoever if I'd ever see him again, and I wasn't completely sure whether that was good or bad, but deep down I thought it was for the best. Our relationship had many ups and downs, and his moods had remained unpredictable. I nevertheless couldn't just disappear. I owed him a telephone call, if nothing else. I threw a quarter into the pay phone inside the terminal and dialed his number. There was no easy way to break the news to him, so I just "put it out there," like an artist who exhibits a picture that may or may not be received very well.

"Darryl, I'm leaving Jackson for a while."

That was a lie to soften his reaction. I never wanted to see Jackson again, and now that I was on the phone, listening to the sound of my own voice burn an important bridge in my life, that included Darryl and my mother.

"What do you mean you're leaving?" he asked. His tone was one of disbelief. In his mind, he owned me, and he wasn't inclined to let his girl get away. "Where are you now?"

"I'm at the Greyhound station. I'm going to Phoenix to live with my sister."

"Why do you need to do that? We can get a place together, you and me. You don't have to move." His tone had transformed from confusion to anger. I was his girlfriend, the one whose every movement he kept track of, the one who wasn't supposed to have other friends. "I'm coming to the station right now—and you better be there when I arrive."

A threat—the kind I'd become accustomed to. The bridge continued to burn.

I took a deep breath and swallowed hard. "Darryl, I won't be at the station when you get here. My bus is boarding right this minute. I just can't do this anymore."

"Listen, Melanie, you—"

I hung up. I didn't want to give him the chance to talk me out of my decision, a decision that I knew in my heart was the right one. The only future I had was in Arizona. I didn't want to be anyone's property any longer.

The announcement that my bus was boarding echoed again through the dirty station. Homeless people slumped in some of the seats, their clothes ragged and worn.

Homeless. Ragged and worn. That was me, even living with my mother or dating an older man who bought me gifts. If I *did* have a home anywhere in the world, it was thousands of miles due west. I boarded the bus.

The trip was bittersweet. As is always the case with the human heart, it looks back, trying to second-guess itself with what-ifs. Would Darryl and I have stood a chance? Not really, but he had been kind to me despite his flare-ups, and for that I was grateful.

And then there was my mother. We weren't on the same page—maybe not even in the same book. She wanted me to be an obedient robot, getting up every day to attend a third-rate high school and live a life of loneliness. But she had given me my letter of dismissal, so to speak, and I could only conclude that she didn't care for me. I supposed that, somewhere deep down inside, she loved me, but she didn't know how to show it. Tonya would hopefully grant me more freedom, allowing me to have friends and a little mobility. She was older, but not so old that she couldn't understand what it was like to be fifteen and want to push established boundaries a bit.

As far as school was concerned, I was behind thanks to the watered-down curriculum at Callaway, but I knew I had what it took to catch up. Academically, I'd do fine.

The bus turned onto the Interstate, and for the next two days, the Greyhound's thick tires rolled across the hot asphalt, taking a full day just to cross Texas. I stared at the passing desert landscape and dozed on and off as people in the back drank or played cards. Stale air hissed through the vents next to every window. If I could have sat in the driver's seat, I would have seen my life in Jackson retreating in the rearview mirror until it was no longer visible.

* * *

I got off the bus, stretched, and walked into the terminal. With her three-year-old daughter Sloane in her lap, Tonya was sitting in an uncomfortable plastic chair that had a small black and white TV attached. For a quarter, passengers could watch fifteen minutes of television while waiting for an arrival or a departure. She and Sloane were doing just that as I approached. She looked up and smiled when she saw me, and after two days on a Greyhound, a welcoming smile is no small thing.

"How was your trip, sis?" Tonya asked.

"Long," I answered. "Long and smelly." The smelly part was why I hugged her tentatively. "I really need a shower."

"Let's get some food and then head back home," Tonya suggested.

That sounded like heaven. Food, a shower, and home.

Was I *really* home? The word itself now held so many connotations for me.

Yes, I thought. I'm home. I'm in Phoenix again, and I'm living with my sister. The tedium and discomfort of the long bus trip were replaced by relief and hope. The city—its buildings, streets, people—was familiar.

Places form indelible memories in our brains, and Phoenix was looking pretty good in the first moments of my homecoming.

Our first stop was at a Circle K so that my sister could get a Big Gulp—sixty-four ounces of Dr. Pepper. Yeah, I was home all right. My sister drank so much Dr. Pepper that I had always teased her that she would end up actually peeing the popular soda.

Next, we hit the streets in the triple-digit heat of Phoenix and found a McDonald's, where I requested an application. I was grateful to Tonya for the chance she was giving me, and I wanted to help in any way possible, and that meant earning a few dollars if I could.

Upon arriving at Tonya's place, I realized how much her situation had changed since her divorce had been finalized. Her one-bedroom apartment, not much more than 450 square feet in size, was cramped and hot. There was no AC, just an electric fan that Tonya had left running while picking me up at the bus station. I'd always thought that there were two requirements for living in Phoenix: air conditioning and a pool within half a mile of my home. The first was obviously not in the offing, but in Phoenix, patches of blue—small swimming pools—dot the landscape in most residential areas of the city. That would be no problem, therefore. The objective was to simply "get wet" on the sweltering days of summer. Even better, McDonald's, assuming they hired me, was just a few blocks away.

I had only been in town for a few hours, but I already felt relieved and happy. Jackson had been a bad dream.

That night (and every night), we slept in Tonya's queen size bed, Sloane happily wedged between us. Sloane's foot often pushed against my back as she squiggled and squirmed, her head sometimes landing near my feet, but I was content for the first time in a long time. I was with people I loved, people I could talk to, and I was relaxed. No walking on eggshells, no snobby kids making fun of the way I talked, no silent mother pretending that I wasn't even in the house.

With school starting in a few weeks, Tonya helped me register in the International Baccalaureate program at North High. The program was designed for gifted students who desired challenging classes that would allow them to earn college credit, as is the case with the Advanced Placement program in most high schools. I briefly wondered if too much time had passed while in Jackson—would I *really* be able to get back into an academic rhythm?—but I knew that I would do well when test time rolled around. I enrolled in English, Math, History, Biology and French.

McDonald's hired me a few weeks later, and I enjoyed the job. I proudly wore my striped shirt, black pants, and cap with burgundy visor as I stood at the first drive-up window, where I simply took orders before cars rolled up to the next window, where drivers grew impatient while waiting for their food. I had landed the plum assignment. No gripes from hungry customers; no complaints about receiving the wrong order. Aside from work, I studied hard and didn't socialize a great deal.

The plum assignment didn't last long. For reasons I didn't understand, the manager moved me to the grill, greasy and hot, where the boys usually worked. The pace was frenetic, and the noise of orders being shouted from one work station to another kept the adrenaline flowing at a steady rate. Personality-wise, I was more of a "customer service" girl, but this was my new assignment. Worse yet, uniforms got dirty with so many patties sizzling hour after hour. To get the brown stains out, I hauled my clothes to the laundromat and sat for a mind-numbing hour and a half while thumbing through a magazine or blankly watching the dryers tumble. One had to be careful. Turn around or walk down to the corner for a snack, and your clothes might be gone when you return. I got frustrated with this routine, so I simply spot-cleaned the uniforms at Tonya's and then wore them again. After a few minutes at the grill each afternoon, no one could really notice when the stains materialized.

Money grew tight as winter approached. Tonya left the oven door open for heat, and I brought home unsold cheeseburgers and fries left under the red lamps near the counter and reheated them for Tonya, Sloane, and myself. The manager didn't care since the wrapped burgers would have otherwise gone to waste. It was the only perk of the job.

I had wanted to become a doctor since my freshman year. I'd always had a keen interest in science—and an aptitude to match—and I was particularly interested in my eleventh grade biology class, which covered a great deal of human anatomy. My mind was set on going into medicine, and I studied hard in Phoenix that year. My teachers inspired me (as I knew they would), and I was once again challenged. I was surrounded by other bright students, and I felt I could do anything. Medicine? Why not? The sky was the limit.

Spring is when the migraines once again hit. I was putting a hundred and ten percent into my schoolwork since I had a definite career goal, but working and helping my sister with Sloane in addition to hitting the books was overwhelming. With so much on my plate, there was little margin for error. Work, school, Sloane—over and over. I didn't mind any of these tasks, but there were only so many hours in a day. When the pain started creeping into the right side of my head, often accompanied by nausea or an aura of light, I couldn't do much of anything. Indeed, whatever I was doing at the moment had to be discontinued immediately. Just as at my grandparents' farm, I was sensitive to light and sound when the headaches came, and the mere anticipation of the next migraine terrified me. Tonya and I had little money and no health insurance, and so my only treatment option was to escape to a dark, quiet room. This absence of sensory input tamed the beast sometimes, but usually the pain intensified since I was left alone with my thoughts. *When is this going to end? Why does it hurt so much? What did I do to deserve this? What if lose my job or can't take finals?*

Unless one has experienced migraines, it's hard to empathize with someone enduring such intense pain. I felt lonely and isolated again. I'd promised Tonya that I would do any and everything to help her when I had pleaded with her to let me move in. Now I was powerless. It wasn't that much different from the summer I went to help grandma after my grandfather died. I was supposed to be the helper, but the stress had laid me low. Years later, the pain was again sapping my ability to contribute to a family household, and my role as caregiver was compromised.

I was preparing for work one day when I felt the onset of yet another migraine, a slight throbbing on the side of my head. It was 1:30 p.m. on a Saturday, and my shift at McDonald's began in thirty minutes. The anxiety and throbbing increased simultaneously with each passing second, and I lay down for ten minutes, hoping that the headache would abate just enough to allow me to make it into work (even though I knew that the killer pain wasn't going away in such a short time). Sure enough, the pain intensified further.

It was now 1:40 p.m. I felt trapped. The worst-case scenario was that I would miss my shift, so I called my manager and told him I was sick. He was a typical twenty-something who enjoyed having power over his teen employees, and I found no sympathy on the other end of the line.

"If you miss work," he said, "you're fired."

Fired? Because I had a headache? I'd never been late for a shift or called in sick—not once. I therefore told him I would be there.

1:50 p.m. I knew I'd be late, but I had to try, hoping the manager would look the other way. I started walking to the restaurant while massaging my right temple, but the bright sunlight was more than my eyes could handle, so I stumbled along, eyelids nearly shut. The trip was surreal—traffic sounds blared in my ears—and McDonald's seemed to recede farther away with each step I took.

It was now 2:05—already five minutes late—and I knew I couldn't get to my job before 2:30. I wondered if I would even be functional if I made it there given the loud chatter behind the counter and the beeping and clatter of the machines. *I'll have a Big Mac and a Coke . . . May I take your order? . . . Who's on register two? . . . A cheeseburger and large fries! . . .*

I slumped onto the bench at a bus stop only three blocks from my home. I leaned over, head in my hands, and cried. I was going to lose my job. Maybe I'd fail my finals, too. The hot Arizona sun beat down on the sidewalk mercilessly until I couldn't stand it anymore. I made my way back to Tonya's and crawled under the covers.

As expected, I lost the job. The manager didn't care about my headaches and had dozens of applications in his desk. Fast food employees came and went. It took me two days to muster the courage to tell Tonya.

I knew that our financial hardship was going to increase. Tonya had worked at several entry-level jobs—lab tech, paralegal, office assistant, and many more—but none of them paid a decent wage. The only silver lining in the dark cloud that had settled over my life was that the migraines tapered off thanks to teachers who were far more understanding than my boss at McDonald's, giving me extra time with finals or postponing them if I didn't feel well on any given day. I did fine, and my next task was to find a new job. Maybe it had all been a temporary setback. It was time for a new game plan, that's all. Maybe the next job would pay more and not be as stressful.

Tonya asked me to watch TV with her after my last final. I looked forward to a little sister-to-sister time since I was feeling better and school was over.

"Melanie," Tonya said as we watched a sitcom, "I've been talking with Dot, and we decided that you need to go back to Mississippi."

My heart sank.

"Back to Mississippi?" Surely I'd heard wrong. "No, I can't. I never want to go back to Jackson. I've already told you—there's nothing for me there. I just need to finish high school in Phoenix. I'm a junior. Things are good for me here. I only have one more year to go!" Tears ran down my cheek.

Tonya and Mom had obviously discussed the migraines and the loss of my job. I had the uneasy feeling that the decision had already been made. It was a *fait accompli*.

"I tried to keep you here as long as I could," Tonya continued, "but things are getting tighter financially, and—"

"If this is about work and money," I interrupted, "I can get another job. Easily. Please don't do this to me, Tonya." I was almost yelling.

I didn't want to be disrespectful to my older sister, but I had to let her know how I felt. All I needed was a few days to land another job. Fast food restaurants were everywhere, or I could do something else entirely. I was willing to do just about anything. How could my sister and mother have made this decision about my life without consulting me?

"I'm going for a walk," I said.

I wanted to slam the door on the way out but resisted the temptation. Neither Tonya nor Mom apparently understood the importance of doing well in high school to ensure being admitted to a good college. It wasn't a priority when they were my age, and they couldn't identify with my plight. I was aware that Tonya's life was tough, trying to support a child after a rocky divorce, but I thought she could have been more sympathetic.

My frustration was amplified by the fact that, despite the migraines, I'd made all As and Bs in my classes. In fact, Mrs. Hawkins, a petite blond teacher I'd been very fond of—early forties—had taken me under her wing since my arrival at North High. She'd been my history teacher and unofficial mentor. Maybe she would have an answer to my dilemma. I called her home number from a pay phone and filled her in on the latest episode of my soap opera existence. I related how frightened I was that my life would fall apart again back in Jackson. I couldn't visualize any future for me there, certainly not one in which I was in control of my own destiny.

Mrs. Hawkins provided reassurance that everything would be fine. She consoled me for half an hour and asked that I call her the following evening.

At home, I was cold to Tonya, offering not a single word of conversation. I fantasized about taking a Greyhound to anywhere but Jackson, although I had no idea how I could take care of myself. The money I'd earned at McDonald's was gone, having been spent on food, bills, and other necessities. A bus ticket to nowhere wasn't a viable option.

I called Mrs. Hawkins the following evening as requested. What I heard was nothing short of astounding.

"Melanie, sweetie," Mrs. Hawkins began, "I had a long talk with my husband, and we both agreed that you can stay with us until you finish high school. We'll even assume legal guardianship, although such a step will have to be approved by your mother and your sister."

"Really?" I asked. "I mean . . . *really?*"

I was shocked but happy. Here was an individual who understood the importance of my medical aspirations. I was a bit guarded at first—it fell under the heading of "too good to be true"—but I took her at her word. My solution had appeared.

"Thank you," I said. "Thank you, thank you, thank you. I'm going to call my mom right now!"

I knew Tonya would be okay with the new arrangement, but everything would hinge on my mother's reaction. I hung up and reached into my pocket for change. It would take a lot of quarters to call Jackson and convince my mom that living with a teacher would enable me to realize my dreams. I fed several quarters into the slot and listened to the phone ring at the other end.

"Hello?"

I could barely contain myself despite knowing the hurdle I was about to meet.

"Mom, I can hardly believe it, but Mrs. Hawkins, my history teacher, said I could live with her and her husband until I graduate. She just needs your permission to—"

"No."

She'd dropped the hammer pretty fast. I didn't even have time to make a coherent argument. I continued anyway, determined to have my say.

"No? What do you mean? Why not? Mom, how can you keep me from such an opportunity? I'm doing great out here. I make excellent grades and am active at North. I intend to run for senior class president, then apply for college and—"

She cut me off a second time. "It doesn't matter what you want. You need to be here. *Here.*"

I stood frozen, my heart skipping a beat. It didn't make any difference what I wanted. It never had and never would. Not wanting her to have the satisfaction of hearing me cry, I hung up before I let the tears flow.

Of course, Darryl was there in Jackson—Darryl, who had written me letters every two weeks, saying he missed and loved me. He'd recounted things we'd done together and wrote that he hoped I wasn't seeing anyone. Until now, I hadn't given his letters much thought since I was hyper-focused on school and work, but now . . . did he still care? I recalled how he had pleaded with me not to leave as I stood at the pay phone in the Jackson bus station. Maybe my absence had made him think twice about the way he sometimes ordered me around. Maybe—just maybe—his temper would subside since he knew I wasn't a "sure thing" anymore.

Maybe.

I called Mrs. Hawkins and told her the disastrous news. I felt bad— bad for her, for me, for my future. She generously told me I could speak to her anytime I felt the need. My intuition, however, told me this was probably going to be our last conversation.

I reached into my pocket again and fished out a few more quarters so I could call Missisippi again.

"Darryl," I said, "I'm moving back to Jackson." I delivered the news as abruptly as when I'd told him I was leaving.

"It's about time you came to your senses," he said. Was I detecting an edge in his voice? A bit of attitude? "When you moving back?" he asked.

"Pretty soon. I have to take the bus, so it'll be a few days."

"You goin' back to Dorothy? Either way, I miss you. Not a day goes by that I don't miss you."

If there had been an edge to his voice, it was gone now. He was the sweet man who had taken care of me. A little warmth crept through my body. I had someone to return to. Hopefully, less controlling.

"See you soon," he said.

"Bye."

* * *

I spent the next day packing, cramming the few items I owned into the same worn suitcase I'd used since eight grade, the same one that had held my life while moving from Jackson to Phoenix. Books, photos, backpack, clothes, make-up, my journals—these were still the meager possessions that helped define Melanie Watkins.

My sister's parting words did not do much to ameliorate the rift between Tonya and me.

"Baby sis," Tonya said, "you know I love you. Maybe one day you'll realize why I couldn't help you out any longer. Anyway, Dot says she's going to try to be more understanding."

The words rang hollow. I had no clue as to why I wasn't being allowed to spend a week or two looking for another job.

"Don't sugarcoat this, Tonya," I shot back. "This has Mom's stamp all over it. She has no understanding at all about my situation. She made that perfectly clear during our last phone conversation, if you can even call it that. I was barely able to get a word in edgewise."

I didn't want to be mad at Tonya, but I was, so I gave her a half-hearted hug. I then kissed Sloane on the cheek and headed for the bus station, which was becoming a grim symbol of my life. I looked back one final time as I left Tonya, hoping that she would relent at the last minute and motion for me to come back. What I got was a wave goodbye from Tonya and Sloane, whose tiny arm was moved back and forth by my sister in a gesture of bye-bye. With tears in my eyes, I walked up the stairs of the bus and sat in the seat directly behind the driver. Placing my pillow against the window, I cried myself to sleep.

The trip back to Jackson was a lot longer than the trip out to Phoenix.

* * *

4

The only redeeming feature in Jackson in June of 1993 was Tougaloo, an African-American college on the northern edge of the city. It offered a summer program for students entering their senior year in high school and who were interested in pursuing careers in science. I was attracted to Tougaloo because it housed students in the summer program on campus—I wouldn't have to butt heads with my mom every day of the week—and it would allow me to meet other kids my age interested in science. The connection with peers who shared my interests had been sorely lacking. The program also represented a foretaste of college, the brass ring I so desperately wanted to grab. It was a win-win situation all the way, although I was far from overjoyed at having to live in Jackson once again. I was accepted into the program and was eager to begin.

As for Darryl and I, we began seeing each other almost before the bus fumes could rise over Jackson and disperse. I anticipated a new beginning in our relationship, and our reunion was a happy one. Our renewed relationship resulted in my becoming a slacker at Tougaloo almost right away. I quickly rediscovered my old habits of sneaking around, trying to beat the strict curfew enforced for high school students in the Tougaloo program. (College students could come and go as they pleased.) My mission had less to do with studying than finding ways to see Darryl. I went out of my way to be nice to everyone on campus who had the slightest bit of authority, even undergrads working in security, as Darryl and I pretended to be students. He and I carried around textbooks and looked like a couple of leisurely coeds going about our business. It was a lot easier than trying to fool my mother, for our subterfuge was conducted in the open.

The program was two months long, and only in the last two weeks did I really apply myself thanks to my chemistry instructor, who was on me like white on rice. He could tell that I wasn't giving his course my all since he was aware that I was one of the brighter students, so he was firm but encouraging as he challenged me to finish all of my classes with hard work and dedication. His concern for me paid off. I won the Most- Improved-in-Chemistry Award, and were it not for this teacher, I probably wouldn't have completed the program. Like Mrs. Hawkins, he demonstrated that there were people who cared about my future and my goals.

That didn't mean I was out of the woods, academically or emotionally. When senior year at Callaway began, I was far more anxious and insecure than I'd been in my sophomore year. My transcript was good despite having moved from city to city in so short a period of time, but I had no idea where I would attend college. Indeed, would I be able to attend *any* college? I nevertheless hoped against hope, knowing all the while that if I did attend college, there was a better than average chance that I might not get into the university of my choice. I knew such an eventuality might well affect whether or not I could get into a pre-med program, but any college would be better than flipping patties on a grill. I'd have to cross that bridge when I came to it.

I'd been embarrassed to set foot inside Callaway again after bragging at the end of my sophomore year that I was returning west, as if I'd been temporarily misplaced and sent to Jackson due to clerical error, and was therefore headed back to civilization. In the midst of such anxiety in my senior year, Darryl was once again my anchor, my constant. Mom didn't really welcome me back, and we more often than not looked the other way if we happened to occupy the same room. We'd picked up exactly where we left off—completely alienated—although now communication itself was held to a bare minimum.

My intimate relationship with Darryl continued as the school year progressed, and little by little I began to test my boundaries again by sneaking out of my apartment at night. Darryl was insistent that I be with him all of the time—no surprise there—and rapidly won me over to his demand that I forsake all other friendships. My mom settled into bed each night by

24

11:00 p.m., and that was my appointed time to peer out the window and look for Darryl in the parking lot of our apartment building. When I felt it was safe, I began my ritual of stepping softly down the steps and out into the night, the cool evening air on my face giving me a sense of liberation. Each time I snuck out, I felt a greater sense of power, growing defiant and bold. The time I was away at night increased incrementally—one hour became two, two hours became five—until I was slipping back in each morning at 5:00 a.m. and crawling beneath my covers, as if I'd been there all night, sleeping like a baby.

On one particular night, Darryl kissed me on the cheek with an affectionate "Hey, baby."

I turned abruptly away, facing the front door of my building. The euphoria and power of escaping each night had turned to guilt, and Darryl sensed the change immediately.

"She don't care about you," he said, as if reading my mind. "She doesn't care if you leave the house or where you go."

Could that be true? I hadn't considered the possibility that my mother was turning a blind eye to my secret forays into the night, indifferent as to my whereabouts. I felt ambivalent, as when Mom had given me permission to move to Phoenix. My eyes filled up as my sense of power ebbed. Maybe my mother had stopped caring for me altogether.

Darryl drove me to Taco Bell, but I couldn't shake the feeling that Mom was sleeping peacefully, unconcerned as to what I was doing.

She don't care about you. She don't care if you leave the house or where you go. The words repeated in my head like a tape loop.

We drove to Darryl's mother's house, which was only five minutes away. He lived with his mom, who appeared to suffer from mild mental retardation. Or perhaps she was just the victim of not getting beyond the sixth grade—I'm not sure—but she had little to say. Quiet, obese, and dark-complexioned, she stayed in her bedroom watching television most of the time, leaving us free to hang out undisturbed in Darryl's room.

Darryl's father was a white man he'd never known, a man much older than his mother. I tried to imagine the scenario from 1971, when Darryl was born, and it was not hard to envision a white man taking advantage of a young, mentally challenged woman of color. In fact, it was probably all too common in the rural south in the sixties and seventies.

Darryl and I went to his room while the TV in his mom's room droned on, filling the small two-bedroom home with unintelligible syllables. Above Darryl's bed hung a large picture of Christ on the cross. Darryl wasn't religious, and I surmised that his mother had hung it there at some point in the distant past. My love of God hadn't changed, but I hated the picture's placement, Jesus always staring at me when Darryl and I made love. I never had the courage to ask him to take it down since my tough, tattooed boyfriend probably did everything his mother asked, and she obviously wanted it there.

"Get me a beer," Darryl ordered, sitting on his bed, opening a bag of nachos.

"Okay."

I wondered why he would order me to do something he could so easily do for himself, but I figured that it was no big deal since he always did so much for me. No, a beer wasn't too much to ask for.

I went to the kitchen, opened a can of beer and poured it in a mug, and returned to the room, where Darryl was already eating the nachos. He took the beer, placed it on the nightstand, and began to touch me as he had done on so many prior occasions, a prelude to sex. I had never refused him, but on this night I felt guilty. I gazed up at the picture, and the sad eyes of Jesus seemed to reflect my own misery and suffering. The Lord was nailed to the cross and couldn't move. In a way, my situation was no different.

"I don't want to," I said. "Not tonight."

"Come on, baby," said Darryl. "You know you want to. What's your problem?"

I shifted my position, feeling uneasy. God, wherever he was, was indeed watching me, and the tape loop of Darryl's words continued to fire the synapses of my brain: *She don't care if you leave the house or where you go.* There were too many ideas to process, too many feelings of inadequacy and guilt.

"I don't know," I said. "I've just got a lot of things going through my mind. I'm just not in the mood."

"You don't have anything to worry about," he said. "You don't work. All you do is go to school. Besides, I take care of everything." His voice grew harsh. "You need to take care of *me*."

Darryl was drinking heavily at this point in our relationship, so much so that he often smelled as if he were sweating alcohol. He was drinking now, and his remarks were condescending: *All you do is go to school. You need to take care of me.*

"I've got to go to the bathroom," I said, standing and heading for the door. I felt nauseous. Darryl grabbed my hand, spun me around roughly, and pulled me towards him, pinning me against the wall. My breathing was shallow and rapid. He'd never done anything like this before. He'd spoken harshly on many occasions, but he'd never become physical.

"When I ask you to do something," he said, "you do it! You understand? You do what I say." He spat out the last three words slowly for emphasis: *What . . . I . . . say.*

As if assenting that his words would always have dominance over my thoughts and actions, I nodded.

Darryl backed up and splashed beer on me with a flick of his wrist. I was too scared to move.

He paused. "I never punched you," he added, a strange non sequitur that seemed, in his own twisted thinking, to cover the harsh treatment he'd just doled out.

""Darryl!" came a voice near the hallway. "Darryl! Is that you?"

His mother walked in, looking disturbed. "What are you doing to that girl?" she asked. "You laid hands on her?" She sounded more annoyed than anything else, as if Darryl had interrupted her favorite game show or sitcom.

"No, ma'am," her son responded.

"I'm taking that girl home," the mother said.

I was never called by my name in that house. To Darryl, I was "baby." To his mother, I was "that girl."

"Come on, girl," she said, addressing me. "I'll take you home. Darryl ain't got no sense."

"Mama," asserted Darryl, "you don't have to do that. I'll take her home."

I most definitely didn't want Darryl to take me home. In fact, I didn't want him anywhere near me. Sitting alone with him in his car? No, not even for a few minutes. I didn't think it was safe to be with him, at least not for the rest of the evening. He'd been drinking, and he might whisper softly and call me his "baby" . . . or, then again, he might continue to order me around, maybe even become physical again.

"Darryl, you ain't no good," his mother said by way of emphasis. "You been drinkin' that al-kee-hall." Her thick southern accent drew out every syllable.

I stood next to the large woman for protection. Darryl never talked back to his mother—that was reserved for me—and she was my only defense during these very tense moments. We exited through the front door, and when she started the car, I told her where I lived. By the time she pulled up to my apartment building, it was midnight.

I approached the door and turned the key in the lock, but the door didn't open. Inside, the chain was on.

Darryl had been correct. Mom knew I'd been leaving at night and didn't care. As for Darryl's mother, she sped away, not waiting to see if "that girl" made it inside safely or not. I sat outside all night, crying. I was alone and couldn't sleep. The once-liberating night air felt harsh and cold.

When my mother opened the door on her way to work the next morning, I apologized to her. She made no reply, nor did she even look at me. She simply brushed past me, the air around her like ice. At least the door was open and I could go inside, take a shower, and get ready for school.

As I slowly shuffled to Callaway, Darryl pulled alongside in his sports car, driving slowly to match the pace of my walking. I looked straight ahead, not wishing to get baited into an argument about the previous evening's events. He pulled a few yards ahead and parked by the curb. Stepping out of the driver's side, he walked towards me holding a single rose.

"You're so pretty," he said. "Why you have such a frown on your face?" He paused. "Listen, I'm sorry."

I should have known better than to expect an argument. Darryl was a manipulator, and an apology was more consistent with his pattern of ensuring that I would remain his "baby."

"Sorry for what, Darryl?"

Was he sorry for his actions or that his mother had intruded upon his abusive behavior towards me. Was he apologizing for spinning me around or for getting caught in the act by a mother who'd proclaimed, "Darryl ain't no good."

"I was mad at you," he replied, "but it won't happen again. We need to be together. This not gettin' along, it ain't right for us." His face softened as he uttered the last words with humility and contrition.

I paused before accepting the rose. The road in life forks with each and every decision we make. I didn't know where I stood with my mother, who probably hated me given that she'd chained the door the previous evening. In front of me, however, was a man who wanted to be with me. It was hard to imagine life without him. If he had a temper or drank too much, then so what? Big deal. I could have had sex with him like I'd done on many other occasions. If I'd given him something so simple, none of this would have happened.

Darryl kissed me on the forehead as I took the rose and lowered my head, staring at its red petals.

"You better get to class," he said. "And do good in school today. I'll pick you up at three."

Controllers are good at covering their tracks, at justifying their manipulative behavior. I once again bought into his sweet, I'm-so-sorry rhetoric and floated on a cloud of relief as I entered the front doors of the high school. As I did so, I positively reveled in the stares aimed at the girl with an employed older boyfriend, a man who had given his baby a rose.

A man who cared about me, whatever his failings might have been.

* * *

5

Mom and I continued our mutual silence over the next few days, our home quiet as a monastery. Feeling sick and nauseated, I stayed in my room most of the time. I think this suited us both. Nothing I could possibly have said was going to thaw the chill hanging between mother and daughter.

Nausea. I wasn't having migraines, but my period was later than usual. I was concerned, but I brushed away the notion that I was pregnant like someone shooing away a fly. My period had never been very regular, and Darryl and I had been careful most of the time, so I didn't think pregnancy was a likely possibility.

Most of the time. Darryl used contraception, but not always. Was he trying to make sure he could "keep" me indefinitely by putting me, as the old cliché goes, in a family way? He'd even pressured me overtly on a few occasions to have his baby, but I didn't want to have a child, not while trying to finish high school and get into college.

Loneliness and alienation can cause the mind to rotate a black and white issue one hundred and eighty degrees until it becomes a murky gray. That's what happened when the word "pregnancy" tried to force its way into my thoughts. My mom didn't seem to care about me anymore, but a needy child wouldn't have a choice. I would care for the baby, and the baby would love me unconditionally. To say that my mother was going to be upset if I turned out to be pregnant would be an understatement, but I wasn't concerned about her reaction. She was Dorothy Watkins, government employee. "Mother" didn't seem to be part of her job description at the time.

The thought of a child loving me and needing me was fleeting. Darryl, however, was elated at the possibility that he might be a father, but his elation frightened me, driving home the gravity of the situation. Pregnant? If that were the case, there would probably be no college and no medical career, only a life with a drunken, controlling man. His on-again off-again tenderness wasn't coming close to covering my fear.

And yet he was all that I had in the way of a constant companion. If I was pregnant, then he was the father. I would have to navigate this difficult situation with Darryl and no one else until I found out for sure if I were carrying a child.

I met Darryl at his home after school the following day. Still elated, he drove me to CVS drug store so we could buy a home pregnancy kit. I hesitated as I walked down the "family planning" aisle where the kits were stocked. There were numerous kinds of at-home tests to choose from, and I wasn't sure whether I should buy a brand name or the store's generic equivalent. If it weren't for the serious nature of my predicament, it might have been laughable that I was worried about thrift at such a time. My entire future was hanging in the balance, and I couldn't even make such a basic decision. Finally, we decided to buy the most expensive kit available because it claimed to be 99.9% accurate. Common sense won out.

The man at the register was a thousand miles distant from my emotional situation. "Are we hopeful or prayerful?" he asked with a smile.

Didn't he see I was a teenager? I responded with a tense, tight-lipped smile.

Darryl and I headed back to his mother's place. Inside, I immediately went to the restroom and opened the kit, a folded leaflet of instructions falling to the floor like a broken accordion. The test required only two drops of urine, which didn't seem like much to render such an important result, but I'd kept my bladder full on the way back from the drugstore, so producing two drops presented no problem.

Technically, my period was not missed, just late, but I stared at the plastic indicator intently. One of two possible symbols would shortly materialize, each one pointing to a different road in life, a different timeline. Would I be a mother? A wife? A student? A doctor? Maybe I'd be all of them. Or maybe I'd be some odd combination of the many possibilities, which wasn't a comforting thought.

Darryl walked in as the positive symbol came into view. He smiled and hugged me, but the intensity of his joy was matched by the intensity of my fear.

"It may not be accurate," I said softly.

Even the most reliable kits carried a disclaimer that a false positive was a possibility. My earlier fantasy of having a child who would need me dissolved into the harsh realities of what motherhood entailed, realities that I doubted Darryl was capable of grasping. I no longer entertained the idea of a soft and cuddly infant in my arms as I stared at the positive symbol again. I didn't want it to be accurate.

"I'll take you to the clinic tomorrow," Darryl said, "but you should be happy."

I felt a mixture of emotions. I was a girl who made good grades and prayed to God. I had good manners and made good decisions—usually. Now I felt like a bad girl. Jesus had seen the whole thing from above Darryl's bed. I was reaping what I'd sown.

The next day, I informed the school nurse that I was sick and had a doctor's appointment. I lied and told her that my older brother was picking me up. There were so many ways of skipping out that I wondered how any school in Jackson maintained attendance. Leaving campus could be as simple as walking away during the change of classes. Regardless, I didn't care if the office called home to confirm that I had an appointment. After all, I was a bad girl, defiant, and I needed to verify the results of the home pregnancy test. If anyone caught me, it was *their* problem.

Darryl picked me up at nine-thirty and dropped me off at the Discovery Clinic, a free clinic a mile from Callaway. It administered immunizations and tested patients for pregnancy and STDs, with no parental consent required for any of its services. Darryl then said he had to leave in order to "take care of some things" and that he'd pick me up at eleven-thirty.

It was hot and humid as it always is in Mississippi in early fall. The clinic, a bare bones facility with no carpeting, music, plants, or tasteful wallpaper, was as warm and humid as the motionless air outside. A fan hung on the wall, its listless blades barely producing a current of air to take the edge off the heat. Near the fan was a poster depicting an unkempt teen holding a crying baby in her lap. The caption read, "Having a baby is like being grounded for eighteen years." I wondered if whomever had put the poster up had considered that, for some patients, such a warning was too late. The message nevertheless had its intended effect on me. Eighteen years was a long time, longer than I'd even been alive. There was nothing in the stripped-down waiting room that gave me any sense of relief.

I signed a fake name—Maria—on the clipboard at the desk and was handed a specimen cup by the receptionist, who told me that the restroom was down the hall. Inside the bathroom was a small window with double doors where a patient was to place the specimen. I left my sample and returned to the lobby to wait my turn. Five other people sat in the clinic that morning, all looking anxious. I wondered what their stories were. HIV? Pregnancy? An STD? Any of these possibilities was more than capable of producing the worried, drawn faces around me.

"Maria?"

Someone was calling my name, and for a split second, I'd forgotten the alias I was using. My mind had wandered while contemplating the grim poster on the wall and the faces of the other patients. I followed a nurse down a corridor to the consultation room. The nurse, a kindly-looking woman, made eye contact with me and said, "Never give up your dreams" as she handed me a slip of paper with the result. I was definitely pregnant.

I'll never forget that comment. It was only five words long, and the nurse probably saw hundreds of people like me every month. She could have remained silent, but she had bothered to inject a ray of hope, as slender as it was, into an otherwise disorienting experience.

My mind was whirling. I was scared, confused, nervous. *A baby will always love you . . . you should be happy . . . you'll be grounded for the next eighteen years . . . never give up your dreams.*

I was finished by eleven o'clock. I sat outside, waiting for Darryl. An hour passed, and I grew worried. Why had he left to begin with? If he wanted a happy family so badly, why wouldn't he want to be by my side every step of the way? By the same token, I was worried that something might have happened to Darryl? Going through pregnancy and birth on my own was a truly terrifying scenario to contemplate.

My thoughts drifted back to my brief visit with the nurse in the consultation room. She'd informed me that my estimated date of confinement—my EDC—was May third. The words from the clinic, printed and spoken, burrowed into my mind. *Grounded. Confinement.* I didn't have much of a social life to begin with, so I reasoned that the only thing worse than being grounded and confined was to be grounded and confined without Darryl.

Darryl pulled up at one o'clock. Having been left alone for hours, I was more than a bit upset. By now, I was worried more about myself and the baby than him.

"Where were you?" I asked.

"You don't need to know where I've been," he answered tersely. "All you need to know is that I've been taking care of important things."

I could tell in an instant that he'd been drinking. For Darryl, that was "taking care of things." He reeked of alcohol.

"So, you still pregnant?" he asked.

The question didn't make any sense? *Still* pregnant? I supposed he was trying to ask if the clinic had verified the home test, but his wording was flippant and uncaring. His enthusiasm had apparently been drowned by alcohol. I didn't make anything of it for fear of setting him off.

"Yes, I'm still pregnant," I said deferentially. "I've had two tests now. It's official."

He had no discernible reaction to the news that he himself had longed to hear, and I was very disappointed at his lackluster demeanor.

"When are you going to tell Dorothy?" he asked. He always referred to my mother by her first name, which I considered to be disrespectful, even if she wasn't within earshot whenever he used her name. Additionally, the question was off-center. Telling my mother was, of course, a major concern, but it would have been nice to hear "Do you want a boy or a girl? What names do you like?"

"I don't know," I said. "I'm scared. Besides, I think she may already know because I've been throwing up a lot. I can't tell her, at least not now."

With little discussion to settle the matter, we decided to have Darryl's mother tell my mom. Given the no-nonsense manner of Darryl's mother, she wouldn't attempt to smooth things over. She'd just come out with it: "Your daughter is pregnant." For Darryl's mother, it would be a matter of one party relaying information to another. She would remain unfazed regardless of my mom's reaction.

Back at Darryl's house, I went into a room by myself. I didn't want to listen to the phone call. After a few minutes, however, suspense got the best of me. I had to face the music eventually.

"Darryl, can you take me home, please?"

His answer could have been predicted.

"You ain't got to go nowhere. My mama is talking to Dorothy. You need to stay here with me."

"I'm not feeling good," I explained.

He was still drunk, and his kindness was not currently on display. Indeed, he wanted me to stay and have sex with him, which was the last thing I felt like doing. I suspect that from Darryl's point of view, he figured that concerns about pregnancy were now moot, so why not indulge even further.

I was emotionally trapped and considered giving in to Darryl's selfish desire. I wanted to get away, to be by myself and rest—maybe reflect on the different paths stretching before me—but I was afraid to go home. Stay, go, stay, go. My mind whirled around like an out-of-control carousel.

Darryl's thoughtlessness morphed into verbal abuse.

"Go home! After all I've done for you, how can you do this to me? You going to just leave me? Walk your ass home!"

It was the liquor talking, but of all days to rake me over the coals, why today, the very day it was confirmed that I was carrying his child? What had I done but be obedient to his every whim, including giving him my body? I had tried to be careful with my words all day. This was my reward. I considered giving into his lust yet again to avoid an unpleasant scene, but his eyes were intense, piercing me with blame. Thankfully, his mother entered at that very moment.

"Darryl, what are you doing to that girl now?"

36

That girl. The girl who was carrying her grandchild.

I asked his mother if she would take me home.

"Don't take her home!" Darryl protested. "Let her walk!" He stomped around, knocking over pictures and books like a child throwing a temper tantrum.

Hadn't we been through a similar scene just a few weeks ago? I thought he'd changed, that he was sorry for his crude behavior. *We need to be together*, he'd said. *This not gettin' along, it ain't right for us*. I'd been wrong. He hadn't changed at all. I was still dealing with a man whose concern was for possessions, not feelings.

Darryl's mother took me to her automobile.

"Don't see Darryl no more!" she warned as we slid into the front seat. "He ain't no good. You better hope you lose that baby." She paused. "I'm going to kick him out when I get back home. Yes I am!"

You better hope you lose that baby.

How could she say something so awful, even if she was mentally slow? She possessed enough of her faculties to have a few especially pointed—and accurate—feelings about her son, but she was apparently oblivious to the feelings of "that girl." I cried, but my tears made no impression on her. She simply dropped me off at the front door and sped away.

The distance from the curb to our apartment door seemed longer than a football field. Every step I took was difficult, as if I were wearing lead shoes. I inserted my key and opened the door.

My mother was sitting at the kitchen table. The house was dark except for a single light hanging over the dining room table, where my mother stared at a glass of clear liquid. I guessed her drink was either vodka or gin.

"Go to your room," she said, not looking at me.

"Yes, mom."

My mother offered only one other comment as I headed up the stairs to my bedroom: "We're moving to Reno."

* * *

6

I'd always been a gifted student, but I didn't even know what state Reno was in. Mom didn't volunteer the reasons for the sudden decision to move, but they weren't very hard to guess. The most obvious, which hardly needed articulation, was that Mom wanted to get me as far away from Darryl as possible, and Reno, which I learned was two thousand miles away and in Nevada, would accomplish that goal nicely.

As horrible as it was to endure Darryl's physical abuse, I'd never told my mother about it. Besides spinning me around and pinning me against the wall, my muscular boyfriend had, as a result of his drinking, grasped me around the throat while in his mother's kitchen one evening, as if he were going to choke me. The incident lasted only seconds, and if had wanted to seriously harm me, he certainly could have, but it was more of a demonstration of his superiority and control—in his own mind, at least—than anything else. Even without knowledge of this event, Mom was an analytical, solution-oriented person, and the logical step was to take one very defiant daughter and remove from her from the older man who'd gotten her pregnant. It wasn't hard to do the math. It was a subtraction problem, or "take away," as they call it in first grade arithmetic. Melanie minus Darryl equaled order.

The "warm fuzzies" weren't Mom's strong suit. She sought results.

I like to think that, despite our extremely tense relationship, my mother cared enough to want me in a different and better environment. There was also, I surmised, the possibility of a better government job in Reno, and with more money, she might be able to improve our overall living situation. This was a simple addition problem: a higher salary plus a different environment equaled the first steps in turning around a situation that had gone from bad to worse. In hindsight, I believe she was correct. A nurturing, supportive personality still wasn't in evidence on my mother's part, but I believe that her intention to secure a better future for me was genuine. Meanwhile, the reality that I was pregnant crystallized more and more with each passing day, but not always in a positive fashion. The move to Reno was a few weeks away—Mom had to finalize her change of employment—so I continued to attend Callaway, where I confided in a pregnant classmate that I, too, was expecting. She was emphatic that I keep this knowledge to myself. From experience, she'd learned that it was hard to be confronted by others or realize that people were talking behind her back. Was this what I had to expect until my delivery date? As I started to show, was I going to become an anathema, destined to be singled out, becoming the subject of gossip? New epiphanies about my situation continued to manifest themselves.

Even a school field trip to the fair drove home the awareness that I was now "different." Our physics teacher wanted our class to see firsthand the effects of force vectors, gravity, rotation, fulcrum points, and other aspects of movement by experiencing the rides at the fair. They were monuments to what textbooks could only allude to. I couldn't go on any of the rides, however, because I was experiencing incessant nausea, plus I didn't want to do anything that would jeopardize the baby. I therefore had to set myself apart—forget about *others* singling me out for the moment—choosing to be an adult while my teen classmates did what came naturally: climb aboard the attractions to get whirled, jostled, and turned upside down by the rides. I was about to be thrust into adulthood and needed to assume the role of someone with advanced maturity and judgment.

I was good at science and saw exactly what aspects of motion the rides demonstrated. What I *didn't* see was the inside of a roller coaster car. I was indeed grounded.

* * *

We arrived in Reno on October 31, 1993 during the middle of my senior year. Without permanent housing yet, Mom and I stayed at a La

Quinta Inn. Wooster High School was across the street, so I was able to get to classes easily and quickly every morning. Even though I was four months along, I wasn't showing yet, and no one at school detected I was pregnant. As for my larger place within the school population, I was the only black student in the senior class, a "fly in the buttermilk," as my grandmother used to say. I could only laugh at the irony of how much my situation had reversed, having attended the all-black Callaway High in Jackson.

The stay at La Quinta lasted about a month while Mom searched for an apartment. It was unpleasant being cooped up with my mother in a small motel room each evening, especially a mother who didn't have a great deal to say beyond remarks of a utilitarian nature, such as comments about laundry, food, or the television. There is such a thing, depending upon the family, as too much togetherness. With Mom, it was a matter of "conversation by necessity," and the tension was so great that a migraine even found its way into the right side of my head on one occasion, a painful reminder that stress remained an integral part of my life.

The poster at the Discovery Clinic had proven all too accurate. I'd been grounded at the fair. At the La Quinta, I was confined and unable to have any real privacy. Grounded and confined. Would the rest of my life be like this? Had I dug a hole so deep that I'd never climb out?

I struggled with many difficult decisions during this period. I didn't want to miss Darryl, but I did on those occasions when my mother seemed particularly insensitive or mean. Before leaving, he'd expressed the desire to help during my pregnancy, but I wouldn't let him. In fact, when I informed him of the move to Reno, he hung up on me, his anger boiling over. Five minutes later, he called me back and threatened to commit suicide since he didn't believe I loved him anymore. He then began to cry. He had a special and devious talent for making me feel guilty. Darryl and I had brief contact while I was in Reno—a few brief telephone calls—and he naturally wanted me to return to Jackson, proclaiming his love for me and desire for us to be a family. Ironically, I think he probably *did* love me in his own selfish way, and if the truth be known, I loved him, too. Love is not rational or analytical; it simply exists, even when a relationship is dysfunctional.

I nevertheless hated the fact that it was Darryl who had made me pregnant. I wanted my baby to have so many good things in life—the things *all* parents want for their children—and given Darryl's drinking, temper, and controlling nature, I doubted that he could provide the kind of life I envisioned for our child. Darryl had pointed out that he would be tied to the baby forever, and while I had to admit that this was a literal and biological truth, I could not imagine being with him again. He wasn't fatherhood material—plain and simple—and I dared to hope that one day I would meet someone who would accept me and my baby, someone who was kind, loving, and respectable. But I had heard someone on television say that, "A respectable guy wants a respectable girl." Was I myself respectable anymore? I believed I was, but this was naturally a confusing time in my life, with everything changing almost constantly: cities, homes, schools— even the very hormones of my body, which had more than a little to do with mood and emotion. There were days, therefore, when I wasn't sure who or what I was. Respectable? I hoped so.

When I reached my four-month mark, I knew that my options had been narrowed to either adoption or keeping the baby. The subject of abortion had been raised in Jackson by a neighbor who was a tech at the local pharmacy. She'd had an abortion and said in so many words that it wasn't as traumatic as people made it out to be. If I wanted to complete my education, she told me, an abortion was the easiest way to accomplish my goal. By the same token, if I wanted to be both a teen mother and a good student, well . . . those were not waters that many girls my age navigated successfully. She went as far as telling me that her life would have been very different—and not for the better—if she hadn't had the abortion. I certainly understood where she was coming from, and I entertained the thought of abortion for a short time before squelching it. My faith in God would never have allowed me to go through with the procedure, and after a while, the mere thought of having an abortion made me feel guilty. There was also the consideration that if I terminated the pregnancy, I might never have the chance to have another baby. Complications could arise, or I might never meet someone who I wanted to be the father of my child.

As a choice, adoption therefore took front and center stage when Mom told my Aunt Bertha about my pregnancy. I didn't want to give the baby to just anyone—the idea of a stranger getting my child, which I would probably never see again because of existing confidentiality laws, felt completely wrong—but Aunt Bertha said she would consider adopting my child. This was definitely an idea worth entertaining since the baby would stay in my family, and Aunt Bertha was a kind woman who was a nurse and had a good job as an registered nurse working the intensive care unit in Kansas City, Kansas. Giving the baby to Aunt B, as I called her, would allow me to go to college and pursue my career goals with a certain peace of mind, knowing that the baby would be well cared for. The idea had even more symmetry considering that Aunt B, who was divorced, had experienced infertility issues. Aunt Bertha would have a baby; I would have a college education.

I felt I had no other avenue to realistically consider. Tonya wasn't an option—she was a single mother whose life was already difficult—plus I still wasn't speaking to her. After all, if she'd allowed me to stay in Phoenix, I would never have gotten pregnant. This wasn't conjecture; it was fact. As for Melvin, my biological father, I'd contacted him to test the waters and see if he had turned his life around and was interested in being more of a father to me, the kind that—hoping against hope—might even consider taking me in. He scoffed at the idea, telling me that "you're just like your mother." I wasn't entirely sure what he meant, although he probably was comparing my quest for a logical solution to my mother's "get the job done" approach to life. Not having spoken to him for over two years, I regretted calling him.

As for my mother's possible involvement, she made it very clear that she had raised all the children she was going to raise and that she was less than thrilled about hearing the pitter-patter of little feet again. Mom worked, and even if she'd been willing to take an active role in helping me raise my child (as many grandmothers do), there was a real danger that she might forever remind me of the mistake I'd made. *It's your baby, Melanie. You did this. I'm trying to help, but you're the one who got yourself into this.*

Having run through all the possibilities, I found myself on a Greyhound to Kansas City to go live with Aunt Bertha at the beginning of the year. I'd only spent two months in Reno, but as the bus carried me to yet another home in January of 1994, I didn't know what the future would bring.

I was turning out to be a human physics experiment in movement: Jackson, Reno, and Kansas City in the space of four months. The Greyhound bus was the smelly carnival ride on which the force vectors of my life were being measured. I knew I had to keep moving—feeling sorry for myself wasn't an option—but I wasn't at all sure what I was moving towards.

* * *

7

Aunt Bertha was my mother's younger sister, a plump, bubbly, light-complexioned woman in her early forties. Her smile communicated exuberance, although her brow was often furrowed. This frequent contrast in her facial expressions reflected the dichotomy of her internal world: concern veiled by cheerfulness. Aunt Bertha was truly a kind woman, but she wasn't always able to grasp the complete meaning of things or express her feelings adequately, and I suspect that these traits often frustrated her. The result was that she could be a bit passive-aggressive at times, although for the most part, she was quite pleasant to be around.

Within a week of my arrival, my aunt took me to the local social services office to help me apply for money that would cover prenatal care, Medicaid, living assistance, and other services that fell under the heading of general pubic assistance. We weren't quite sure what we might be eligible for, but we nevertheless sat for hours in the lobby of the government building, waiting to see what resources might be allocated for our particular living situation. We took a number—162—and sat among the other applicants, who represented young, old, black, white, Hispanic, male, female, and the disabled. It was an even mixture of people expressing hope, frustration, fatigue, or resignation to the system. If anyone had told me years earlier in Phoenix that I would one day end up in such an office looking for public assistance, I wouldn't have believed it.

Our number was finally called, and we made our way to a booth where a glass partition separated us from the social worker. The divider spoke volumes about the government's attitude towards those seeking its help. Secure, protected workers were on the "inside," the arbiters of people's fate.

We were quite literally the outsiders, hoping to see what crumbs fell from Uncle Sam's table. My aunt gently slid the application we'd filled out beneath the partition and nodded politely to the woman. I sat as my aunt began talking.

"Good morning," said Aunt Bertha. "My niece is now living with me. She's seventeen and pregnant and will therefore need some assistance. I'm her legal guardian." My aunt's tone of voice revealed the undercurrent of uncertainty I'd noticed in her personality, and it was natural that it would be expressed while negotiating with the juggernaut federal system, although her manner was forthright and honest.

"How many people are in your household?" queried the social worker, not bothering to make eye contact as she held a pen poised over the page, waiting for a response.

"Normally there's just me," Aunt B answered.

The social worker looked up, a puzzled expression crossing her face. "It's just you? You don't have a husband or children?"

"No, I don't," my aunt replied, her voice softening.

"That must be lonely," the social worker said matter-of-factly, looking back down at the application.

The comment seemed insensitive in the extreme, especially coming from a woman who surely saw hundreds of people a day, many of them living alone and down on their luck. For that matter, millions of people who *don't* need to apply for assistance live by themselves. Had the woman become so desensitized by her job that such stray remarks rolled off her tongue each day from behind the partition?

The remark had a secondary consequence, however, one that caused me to reflect more closely on my own situation. After I gave birth, Aunt Bertha would no longer be alone anymore, which was ideal for her, but where would that leave me? Years down the road, would I be the one saying, "Just me?" It was a sobering thought.

The social worker continued our interview, asking about my educational background, Aunt Bertha's employment history, her salary, street address, and other questions that boiled down to routine statistical information. After she'd filled out the necessary paperwork, the social worker said we would hear something from the office within thirty days.

Afterwards, Aunt Bertha took me to the grocery store, filling the cart with all of my favorite foods and asking me what I would like her to cook for dinner that evening. This was heaven, especially after sitting in the grim government office, which just as soon be labeled the Department of Lack and Gloom. Aunt B's offer made me feel special, not something I was accustomed to, and for the first time in a long time, I thought that things might work out for the best. This notion was further reinforced when my aunt, a very good cook, put wonderful meals on the table, dishes such as Cornish hens, turkey, stuffing, macaroni, green beans, mashed potatoes, and so much more. It felt so great to be taken care of for a change. My aunt's TLC went a far way to assuage, even if only partially, my feelings of doubt and lack of respectability.

* * *

Aunt Bertha and I had already visited the mainstream high school, Wyandotte, where the counselors directed us to the Louisa M. Alcott Teenage Mother School, or "TAMS". The Wyandotte counselors advised us that I would feel more comfortable among other young women in my "situation." Additionally, we were told that the TAMS' staff was more experienced in dealing with students who weren't feeling well, missed tests, submitted late homework, or needed to miss school for doctors' appointments.

The Monday after our visit to social services, therefore, my aunt and I walked through the door of TAMS for the first time. At five and a half months, I was quite obviously pregnant. I immediately felt as if I didn't belong there. The students were my age, and some were even farther along in gestation that I was, but they looked distant and distressed, as if they had no spirit left, no dreams. Many of the girls were on their second pregnancy, and the school struck me as a juvenile facility. The despondent atmosphere was palpable.

Aunt Bertha and I approached the counter.

"This is my niece Melanie," Aunt B said. "She's pregnant and we need to register her for school."

The secretary handed us a clipboard and requested that we complete the registration paperwork (which I'd already had quite enough of thanks to the many forms at social services). Thankfully, my aunt filled out the information while I sat next to one of the pregnant girls. I turned my face slightly, trying not to stare. The teenager leaned over, head in her hands, elbows on her knees. She was the essence of frustration and fatigue, and I didn't want to be around such people. Since my early days in Jackson (and excluding my stay in Phoenix), I'd had to endure the company of students who I could not emotionally or intellectually relate to, and it appeared that I was now taking another step down. I didn't want to be sequestered with students whose only goal was day-to-day survival. From what I could see during my initial visit, TAMS gave off the quintessential bad vibe. As I would do more and more frequently, I began to rub my belly since the gentle, circular motions of my hand on my abdomen helped me feel grounded when everything around me was surreal. Inside my body was a baby, someone who relied on me for life, and this knowledge was a comforting reality when stress tried to overtake my thinking.

After Aunt B returned the clipboard, the secretary informed us that classes were only scheduled for half a day so that the students could address whatever came up. Each pregnancy was different, and the students at TAMS needed built-in time to deal with health issues as they arose. The secretary also stated that every girl had to take child development and nutrition courses. Finally, we were told that there was one counselor for all of the students: Miss Berry.

The presence of single counselor wasn't a good omen. If the needs of the institution's population were diverse enough to warrant cutting the school day in half, didn't TAMS need more than one person to help with emotional crises, not to mention college applications? How could one counselor handle the needs of students who looked to be the very definition of sadness and defeat?

"Is Miss Berry available?" I asked.

"She's with another student, and that student right there—" She motioned to a girl in a nearby chair. "That girl is waiting to see her as well."

We thanked the secretary, and my aunt and I said our goodbyes. It was time for me to take over from there—time to assume the role of adult, as I'd learned at the fair. It was my first day of class.

I walked into the child development classroom, where the eyes of ten other students shifted toward me.

"Um, hi. I'm Melanie Watkins, the new student."

"Here's your textbook," the teacher said. "Have a seat, please. We're on chapter two."

The desks were roomier than normal high school desks in order to accommodate those students who were farther along than others. The carpet was old, and the facility was essentially a converted house, an extension school for the mainstream Wyandotte. Feeling totally out of place, I sat through a lecture on what a uterus was. My heart sank—how far down could it go?—when I realized that some girls actually didn't understand the basics of their anatomy or the changes their bodies were experiencing.

One of the students approached me after the bell rang.

"My name's Jessica," she said. "When are you having your baby?"

"My due date is May third," I replied.

"You have a name for it yet?" she asked. "Mine is going to be Trey. I'm expecting him in two months."

Jessica sounded very sure of herself, as if the whole of her life had been satisfactorily mapped out. I wondered briefly how many girls at TAMS had dozens of details worked out, details that hadn't even occurred to me.

"No," I said. "I don't have a name yet. Actually, my aunt is going to choose a name since she's going to adopt him."

Jessica stared at me in disbelief. "That's stupid!" she said rudely, her face scrunched into a frown. "Why would you carry a baby for nine months and then just give it away? It's your baby. Don't you want it?"

I resented the question, one that was utterly simplistic in nature. Of course I wanted the baby, but there were other factors to consider.

"Well, I want to go to college," I replied, "and I think that might be hard to do while trying to care for an infant. My aunt always wanted a baby, so I thought I would let her adopt it."

The girl remained incredulous, rolling her eyes. To Jessica, I was apparently some kind of strange alien life form. I'm not sure what was more displeasing to her: the fact that I was giving my baby to my aunt, or that I was doing so to attend college. In later days I would learn that virtually all of the girls at TAMS were planning to keep their children and find jobs. It was a simple, basic plan, but not one that meshed with my own thinking. Jessica walked away, unable to fathom my decision. The girl in The girl in Jackson, who'd confided in me that she, too, was pregnant, had warned me about being singled out or talked about. Would I now have to worry about being singled out because I had the audacity to want a college education? It seemed ludicrous, even hypocritical, to think that such criticism would come from other girls who were pregnant and going through a rough patch in their lives, and I had to remind myself that their planned futures and mine were diametrically opposed.

So much for making a new friend on the first day.

* * *

I walked to the office to see Miss Berry the next day. The secretary waved me down the hallway to her office. Miss Berry was a thin black woman with short, cropped hair that accentuated her cheekbones. I introduced myself, after which the counselor motioned for me to sit.

"What can I do for you today, Melanie?" She leaned forward across her desk, body language that indicated she was eager to hear whatever was on my mind, but her tone of voice quickly persuaded me otherwise.

"I'd like to go to college," I said in answer to Miss Berry's question. "I know I'm pregnant, but I'm thinking that I may not be taking the courses I need to get into a good college. Is there any way I can take classes other than child development or nutrition?"

Miss Berry expressed not the slightest bit of interest in my goals. Her reply to my questions was as utilitarian as anything my own mother might have said.

"Every girl at TAMS takes child development and nutrition," Miss Berry began. "How are you going to learn to take care of your baby? And besides, honey, this is a reading, writing, and 'rithmetic school. We just want to see you graduate, dear. That's all you have to do: show up for classes and graduate. Now then, is there anything else I can do for you today?"

The question was phrased to express concern, but it was delivered in such a manner as to shut me up as quickly as possible.

College? What on earth can this girl be thinking about?

"No, Miss Berry. Thank you."

It was now patently evident that TAMS was a babysitting service for pregnant teens. True, they offered two classes that many students would need in order to take care of their children, as well as their own bodies, but that was the extent of the school's educational concerns for its students beyond basic literacy. The future of students at Teenage Mother School was not even a secondary consideration to the staff, including Miss Berry, who, of all people, should have been capable of showing a little empathy for the girls. Wasn't that her job?

I looked upward, hoping God could provide an answer to my dilemma. The word "college" wasn't on anyone's radar at TAMS, a fact that seemed nonsensical. Didn't every graduating senior in the country have the right to basic advice, plus the necessary paperwork, for applying to college? Was my request so unreasonable?

I had nutrition class in five minutes. I hoped that God would at least help me hold back my tears.

I was frustrated, but I was equally determined to find a solution. With TAMS ending in the middle of the day, I decided to take a bus to Wyandotte that afternoon. I called my aunt and told her that I was going to find a new counselor, and she gave me the green light to make the journey after my scheduled classes.

Wyandotte seemed larger than the average high school—or maybe it just *seemed* bigger because the task before me was itself quite big. Students stared at me as soon as I entered the door, a few even pointing and whispering as I approached the front desk. Would I have to endure this same judgment–oriented gaze until I finally delivered? I was beginning to feel like an exhibit on the fairway at an old-fashioned carnival.

"I need to see a counselor," I said. "I'm a student at TAMS."

"TAMS has a counselor," said the secretary, adjusting her glasses in order to see who was making the request. "Her name is Miss Berry."

"I know that," I said. "I already spoke with her, but I'm attempting to apply for college, and she doesn't have any information on scholarships or college admissions. May I talk with a counselor here?"

It's hard to be a high school senior given the many career decisions that need to be made as one moves from adolescence to adulthood. Being a pregnant college senior was even harder. Was I expected to forfeit my dreams because of my pregnancy?

"The counselors here are busy with their own students," was the secretary's curt reply. "This is a very busy time since our seniors are applying for college."

This answer was really hurtful. I thought of other activities that accompany one's senior year: proms, class ring ceremonies, and senior trips, to name just a few. I was jealous of people I didn't even know, but I had come to Wyandotte on this particular afternoon with a purpose, and I wasn't going to be deterred because I was outside Wyandotte's mainstream population.

"I know that your seniors are applying for college," I said, "but I need to start applying, too. I'm adopting my baby out to my aunt, so I'll be able to attend college this fall."

I added the statement about adoption since the secretary was looking at me as if it were preposterous for a pregnant teenager to even consider going to college. I was meeting resistance from pencil-pushers and insensitive people wherever I went, whether I was seeking Medicaid or college admissions information.

The secretary reluctantly picked up a phone and talked to someone briefly. Upon hanging up, I was told I could see a Miss James, one of

Wyandotte's guidance counselors. The secretary pointed to a door a few feet away.

I found Miss James' office after entering a corridor on the other side of the door. At last I'd found someone who was sympathetic to my plight. Miss James was immediately receptive to my requests and was generous with her time, asking me what type of college I'd like to attend. She gave me scholarship applications and discussed admissions tests, letters of recommendation, and admission requirements. I was also reassured that I would graduate with all of the required credits to move forward with the applications process. I held the forms close to my chest as I smiled and left Miss James' office. It was a case of "mission accomplished."

Fortunately, the world has good people, people who take an interest in students fighting the odds, people like Mrs. Hawkins and my chemistry professor at Tougaloo—and now Miss James. I was also learning that I had to be polite but insistent in my quest for the life I wanted, not taking "no" for an answer. I was not going to be grounded or confined, nor was I going to accept the prevailing mindset at TAMS: mediocrity. I had traveled many miles on buses in order to find a meaningful, stable life, and I was determined to make each one count.

My own efforts notwithstanding, maybe God had indeed answered my prayer made earlier that day. I never stopped believing he was looking out for me.

* * *

8

We were approved for Medicaid the following week, and as expected, part of the government assistance included prenatal care. This was during the Clinton administration, when healthcare reform was starting to be seriously debated; with no real changes in place, however, it would be necessary in the coming months to jump through more bureaucratic hoops in order to claim our various benefits. This added to the stress, but at least we were getting help.

Aunt Bertha took me for a prenatal exam at Providence Hospital. At five and a half months, I still didn't know the sex of the baby, but my main concern was naturally to ensure that the baby was healthy and developing normally. On my own, without anyone else's knowledge, I had gone to the Emergency Room of another hospital because my natural instinct was that expectant mothers needed some form of medical care. My growing tendency to act like an adult told me that I might bypass a good deal of red tape by going to an Emergency Room, where a doctor would have to see me. The staff at the ER discovered no problems after a cursory exam, but neither did they provide a great deal of information. I was not, after all, a bona fide emergency. In retrospect, my visit to the ER represented a responsible decision, albeit one that skirted the truth of why I was there, but it also indicated that I was developing a strong maternal instinct.

The exam at Providence General was going to be the real deal. The waiting room at Providence provided a sharp contrast to The Discovery Clinic in Jackson and its grim décor. The beige and mauve-colored waiting room had magazines such as Pregnancy and Parenting on a table surrounded by chairs and flanked by comfortable sofa. I chose the sofa, Aunt

Bertha sitting across from me in a chair. I was coming into contact with many people—teachers, counselors, nurses, and secretaries, who, for the most part, performed their jobs with an assembly line mentality—and I was becoming astute at reading people's body language and vocal inflections. Aunt Bertha was certainly not in the same category as uncaring social workers or secretaries, but I detected her trademark discomfort lurking beneath the surface of a kind, polite demeanor. I am fairly sure she chose not to sit next to me because of her prior infertility issues. I was the one who could feel the baby kicking, the one who was directly connected to my unborn baby by an umbilical cord. Aunt B's physical connection to the child was still months away. Her feelings were totally understandable.

Leafing through one of the magazines, I saw articles on what kinds of prenatal tests expectant mothers should request, as well as pieces on possible complications older women could expect during pregnancy. Given my inquisitive nature, I wondered about what kinds of complications and risk factors younger mothers might encounter. Indeed, what types of tests, if any, were already too late to receive? With the magazine fueling my anxiety, I placed it on the table and sat quietly, as did Aunt Bertha.

And then it was time.

"Melanie?" the nurse announced.

I stood and stepped forward, expecting Aunt Bertha to follow me, but she remained seated. As a nurse, she knew all to well what tests I would receive, and the prospect of getting close to the sights and sounds of the baby was obviously painful for her.

The woman who'd called my name introduced herself as a medical assistant and then asked me to step on the scale. My weight registered at 210 pounds. I couldn't believe it! I was around 150 when I became pregnant. I wasn't sure how much I should weigh at this point, but I was fairly certain that I was carrying too many pounds as a result of Aunt Bertha's home cooking.

I followed the assistant to another room and sat on an exam table. To my right was a large mirror that revealed someone I hardly recognized. I had not been afforded this view before, but now that my image was just a few feet away, I thought myself to be way too large. My face was puffy, my arms looked swollen, and my bottom filled the entire space at the end of the exam table. With my hair in braids courtesy of one of Aunt B's friends (to spare me the trouble of doing my hair), the person staring back at me from the mirror looked like a stranger. I literally didn't recognize myself. Where was Melanie?

It was around this time that I couldn't tolerate mushy boy-meets-girl love stories on television. I couldn't project myself into these shows, feeling that my life would never live up to the romantic plots, most of which contained passion and happy endings. Who would want to be romantically involved with a puffy, swollen woman weighing 210 pounds? A knock on the door interrupted my brief reverie.

Dr. Quinn, one of the staff OB/GYN doctors, entered the room, took a seat on a brown circular stool, and wheeled his way over to me. He was a kindly man who proceeded to ask the all of the pertinent medical questions.

"You're new to our office, correct?" he said. "What was the date of your last menstrual period? Also, have you had an ultrasound yet?"

Which question was I to answer first? I told him that I was indeed new to the office but that as far as my menstrual period was concerned, I could only give him my "best guess" since my periods had never been regular. I told him that I'd never had an ultrasound before or a real prenatal visit, only an initial exam at the clinic in Jackson that had administered the formal pregnancy test. Out of embarrassment, I didn't tell him of my solo visit to the ER a month earlier. He asked further questions about my medical history, and I answered them as best as I could.

"Can I find out if the baby is a boy or a girl?" I asked.

"You'll be scheduled for an ultrasound within a few days," Dr. Quinn answered. "For now, I want to check the baby's heart rate."

I was mortified by all of my stretch marks as he helped me lie down on the exam table—cocoa butter and prayer hadn't stopped them from forming—but I figured he'd seen more than his share of stretch marks while examining pregnant women. The gel he applied to my abdomen was cold, but I smiled as soon as Dr. Quinn located the baby's heartbeat. At that age *in utero*, a baby's heartbeat is fast, sounding like that of a hummingbird's, thumping along at a hundred miles an hour. I'd felt the baby kick before, but now I could hear actual sounds of life, and the sound I was now hearing was the most important sound of all: the heartbeat, which meant that the baby was alive and growing. Inside my womb, a new life was preparing for its entrance into the world. In an instant, the baby became more real to me than at any time in the past.

I scheduled my next appointment, rejoined Aunt Bertha, and headed for the door. That evening, I wrote a poem in my journal. My journal was like a friend, someone who would listen each night to my words and emotions, conflicts and questions, hopes and doubts. In some ways, perhaps I was talking to myself, or then again, maybe I was talking to God. Regardless, the pages over time seemed alive. Every journal, once its pages were filled, was a part of my life, breathing, whispering, reflecting. The poem I wrote that night was about the ultrasound test.

Listening to my baby's heartbeat
Is like listening to the horses galloping in the fields
Running free
I wish we could be free
Be free like runaway horses
That never, ever look back

I wanted my baby to be forever free and unconfined, having a sure path in life that provided enough security so that it would not have to look back or experience regret. I wanted that for myself as well. Indeed, at this time, my baby and I were still one.

Was adoption the right choice? Doubts appeared in my thinking, like a small crack in a pane of glass, a crack that begins to run, growing longer with time, until it is a line etched across the surface of a window. The question from the girl at TAMS echoed distantly in my mind: Why would you carry a baby for nine months and then just give it away?

I pushed the question from my mind. The arrangements had been made.

* * *

Two days later, the TAMS shuttle, always "on call," took me to my ultrasound appointment, the driver promising to pick me up when the procedure was through. This appointment was for the "formal ultrasound," which would not only image the baby but hopefully reveal its sex.

The radiology department was in the basement of the hospital, where I didn't have to wait very long, a welcome relief after having to put up with so my "systems," bureaucratic in nature, in which I had to take a number or compete against my peers for attention. The imaging tech took me inside the dark ultrasound room, with only the dim light of the machine casting a soft glow on the surroundings. I was excited. On my previous visit, Dr. Quinn had told me that the test about to be administered would provide information on the size of the baby, how far along the pregnancy was, details about the baby's anatomy, and the gender—hopefully.

The ultrasonographer, who had a wide smile on his face, looked to be in his twenties—not unusual for a tech—but perhaps he just looked young for his age. Either way, I hoped he knew what he was doing. In the space of a few short minutes, I was about to receive more information about my baby—it was still *my* baby, wasn't it?—than I'd received in the past five and a half months. He applied cold gel across my abdomen and then proceeded to pass a palm-held instrument across my skin so that the sound waves could locate the baby.

I couldn't hold back the question any longer. "Is it a boy or a girl?"

He narrowed his eyes and studied the ultrasound machine, part of which resembled a small black and white TV monitor. "It looks like . . . it's . . . ah, here it is. I see it." He pointed to a white cylindrical shape on the image. "It looks like a penis."

"Wow, it's a penis!" I joked. I asked him for a picture, and he printed out three copies right then and there. These are the first pictures almost every parent receives of a child. One of the printed black and white images had a large arrow pointing to the cylindrical shape, with the word BOY next to it.

The most obvious question had been answered, but not necessarily the most important.

"Does everything look okay?" I asked, straining to keep my eyes on the monitor.

"The radiologist has to make the final report, but I don't see anything that stood out," he replied, emphasizing the last two words.

Was this radiology humor? Nothing "stood out"? Did that mean he'd seen a few unusual things, but either wasn't sure what they meant or wasn't at liberty to discuss them since he was only a tech? Was I going to receive a phone call from the radiologist, who would say, "Miss Watkins, I'd like to see you again to discuss 'a point"?

I decided not to borrow trouble and brushed away the concern. I thanked the pleasant young man and used the phone to notify TAMS that I was ready for the shuttle.

While waiting for my ride, however, I had an uneasy feeling of a different kind. My baby's gender was male. What would I do with a boy? For that matter, how would Aunt Bertha handle a rough-and-tumble boy? Was an older single woman capable of handling a boy who might be the proverbial handful, especially when his hormones kicked in? There would be no mother-daughter bond, and it was not likely that Aunt B would remarry. I had assumed my baby would be a girl, perhaps just wishful thinking on my part. My doubts about adoption returned, and they were stronger than before. Maybe I should keep the baby. A black boy needs a man in his life, and maybe Darryl and I could make it work.

Maybe, maybe, maybe. My head was spinning as the shuttle lumbered up to the curb and I awkwardly made my way to a seat.

What was I going though all this for? What was my goal?

I wasn't sure anymore. Having seen my baby, my world had been tilted on its axis.

* * *

9

One thing that hadn't changed while living in Kansas City was my hope for a college education. I received a letter from the University of Nevada, Reno accepting me into the fall, 1994 freshman class. Miss James had continued to help me, reviewing my applications and discussing plans on which college was the best match for me. Several possibilities had presented themselves, and they were narrowed to two. I was also accepted to Tougaloo, the traditionally black college in Jackson where I had attended a summer science enrichment program in June of 1993 after returning from my brief stay with Tonya.

The reason I'd applied to these two colleges can be summed up in two words: familiarity and finances. I'd first heard of UNR's low-cost tuition while at Wooster High during my very brief stay in Reno at the end of 1993. As for Tougaloo, it also offered significant financial support, with the possibility of a full scholarship—all tuition and expenses paid for top students. As someone who'd grown up without much money circulating in my household, the decision to apply to these schools was relatively simple from a financial point of view. I was also familiar with both cities. Mom was in Reno, although I didn't know what attending college in the same city where she lived would be like. Darryl, of course, was in Jackson, a city I knew all too well, but I was leaning towards UNR. Its program seemed will suited for me, not that I was necessarily counting on Mom's help should I move back to Reno. But anything was possible, and a part of me wondered if she might one day have a change of heart.

* * *

Aunt Bertha was changing, or so it seemed to me. Perhaps sensing my brewing state of ambivalence about whether or not to keep the baby, she became uncharacteristically nice after my second ultrasound. As she lavished me with food and presents, I felt as if she was fattening me up for the kill, like the children in *Hansel and Gretel*. Was she buying the baby, even if only on an unconscious level? In discussing the future of the child, Aunt Bertha stopped short of saying that my identity as the birth mother would never be revealed, but she made it abundantly clear that co-parenting was not part of our arrangement. She was going to be the mother, and her decisions about the child's welfare and upbringing would not be open to question. I seriously doubted that my baby would ever know the truth.

These were unsettling thoughts, and they continued to multiply. Was I emotionally strong enough to listen to the baby calling her "mommy" and me "Melanie"? And if simple utterances could potentially cause me such pain, how would I feel when Aunt Bertha nursed my child through an illness or took him to his first day of school? During all of the milestones in my child's life, I would look at my aunt with envy, knowing that I was the one who deserved to be standing in her shoes.

Old thoughts also resurfaced at this time. What if I were not able to have another baby in the future? What if I decided at some point that I wanted to be with Darryl again? This latter scenario didn't seem likely, but my thoughts revisited all possibilities as Aunt B continued to act as if I were living in a gingerbread house. After all, Darryl wasn't aware that arrangements had been made to have my aunt adopt his baby. It was his biological child, and I wondered with more than a little apprehension what his reaction might be if he learned of my plans. What could he do? More to the point, what *would* he do? Would he take out his anger on me, throwing me across the room in a drunken rage, or would he walk along side me, using his charm?

It just doesn't seem right, Melanie. Me and you have a baby. We're a family. Don't I have a say in all this?

People change. Maybe Darryl had already turned his life around, or at least might be willing to do so upon learning of my present plans for our baby.

Our baby. Yes, it was ours.

* * *

Aunt Bertha invited her best friend Joyce and Joyce's two children, Dante and Erika, to dinner one evening. The night would turn out to be one of the low points of my stay with my aunt. The kids were spoiled beyond belief and had no manners whatsoever. Their mother gave them free rein to say or do whatever they wanted. After dinner, they sandwiched me on the sofa.

"Do you have a husband?" the nine-year-old Erika asked. I don't know whether the question was prompted by my age or by the fact that no male was to be seen in the house.

"No, I don't," I responded, annoyed by the forwardness of the query.

"You're supposed to have a husband if you have a baby," Erika continued.

I took a deep breath and made no further reply. I didn't want to be lectured to by a child.

"Yeah, that's right," Dante offered, "or your baby ain't real." He paused. "So your baby ain't real." The smug attitude of this seven-year-old was offensive.

"Well, then you don't have to touch my unreal baby after he's born!" I blurted out.

I hated the thought of either of these two urchins being anywhere near my baby after he was born, but once Aunt Bertha adopted him, I wouldn't have any say-so in the matter. It was one more fact that added to my growing misgivings about adoption.

Doing dishes in the kitchen, Aunt B must have overheard the conversation. She walked into the living room a few moments later.

"Oh, you just never mind all that," she told me. "Junior will be just fine."

My aunt had started calling my unborn child "Junior," a reference that irritated me. Junior was inside Melanie Watkins, not Aunt Bertha.

Aunt B, Joyce, and the kids continued to talk about the baby. I felt out of place in a room filled with people having a conversation in which I wasn't included. All of the references to my baby were made as if I weren't present, making me feel like nothing more than an incubator. I once again rubbed my belly to soothe myself. I needed to touch my abdomen to prove I still existed. I thought that if the ongoing conversation continued much longer, it might totally eliminate me, causing me to disappear altogether.

After an excruciating hour of their speculation about Junior's future—no mention was made of me, his incubator—I excused myself and went to my room. It was a little girl's room, with a bright pink comforter and lace curtains. Dolls rested on the nightstand. Although the room had a lounge chair that enabled me to tilt back and rest my feet, I understood deep-down that the room had been prepared for the baby. I was its current occupant, but I knew that the soft, lacy trappings had been provided to help me feel calm and relaxed so as not to create any stress for Junior. My aunt was creating an entire world for the baby, complete with plans for its future, a future I would only see glimpses of depending I was given, probably limited, to my child. I was never comfortable in that room again because I realized that its very lovely appointments had not been meant for me.

Given the status quo, what would happen in just a few weeks? After the delivery, I thought it a certainty that I would be pushed farther out of the picture. I would become virtually invisible.

I wasn't at all sure I'd made the right decision.

* * *

I'd had enough of being pregnant by April of 1994. I was large and uncomfortable, but I was also diagnosed with preeclampsia, a pregnancy-related condition characterized by high blood pressure and protein in the urine. The condition can occur in the third trimester and cause the mother to have seizures, which naturally have the potential to affect the baby. I was sentenced to bed rest for the duration of the pregnancy. The only redeeming feature I found of still being pregnant (and being on bed rest) is that it afforded me time to feel close to my baby before giving him up for adoption. Otherwise, bed rest was an exercise in boredom. The doctor recommended a low-sodium diet, which my aunt misinterpreted as a no-sodium diet. Aunt B's once sumptuous meals became bland.

The same could be said for living at Aunt Bertha's house in general. I was a means to an end. I no longer felt special or wanted. Life there had become unappealing.

* * *

10

There were times when life made no sense at all when I was seventeen, as if I were Alice in Wonderland, who'd fallen down the rabbit hole. Every time I thought I had a grasp of reality, the surreal would impose itself. Aunt Bertha left a note for me on the dining room table one morning after she'd left for her 7 a.m. shift. I was dumbfounded when I read it.

Your mother called. She wants you to call her ASAP.

I'd had no contact with Darryl or my mother for five months, two people who had betrayed me and who I felt I could never trust again (except on those occasions when Aunt Bertha's altered behavior caused me to explore the nebulous worlds of "what-ifs"). I picked up the note, but just as quickly dropped it, so that it fell back to the table. I was getting used to life without a mother. I didn't miss her, nor did I feel guilty about my lack of emotional attachment to her.

But what could she possibly want?

I was due in two weeks. My thoughts were completely focused on having the baby and attending UNR in the summer. Besides being enrolled in UNR's fall class, I had been accepted to the Howard Hughes Medical Institute Scholars program on the UNR campus, a course of study for minorities and women interested in math and science careers. The program required that I live in the university dorm, which would be a welcome change from staying in the frilly room prepared for Junior. I was eager to move forward with my education, especially since I felt that I hadn't learned much of anything during the past five months. TAMS was bad enough, but TAMS on bed rest was a joke.

It was at this time, my mind utterly preoccupied with giving birth and starting college, that my mother chose to resurface. Did she have cancer? Did she need to tell me something about Darryl? The latter seemed unlikely given her complete disapproval of my ex-boyfriend, but whatever the case, I needed to know the reason behind the brief, cryptic note on the table. Part of me wanted to show her that not only did I not miss her, but also that I didn't need her—and never would. Nevertheless, I felt compelled to call her in case there really was something seriously wrong, such as a terminal illness. I was bitter, but that didn't mean that my conscience had gone AWOL. It was a grim task I would have to shoulder. I picked up the phone the next day and dialed her number.

"How are you doing, Melanie?"

My mom's voice. Distant yet familiar. The voice that had abruptly sent me to Phoenix and then summarily summoned me back to Jackson. The voice that, for hours at a time—even days, had chosen to remain completely silent when I'd last shared an apartment with my mother.

I forced myself to concentrate on the voice now coming through the telephone. It was uncomfortable yet comforting, a classic case of "hope springs eternal" on my part. Was my mother growing soft as my due date approached? I knew she'd been speaking with Aunt B on the phone to receive updates on how things were working out, but I never learned what details might have been discussed about my pregnancy, TAMS, or the living situation in my aunt's household. I didn't want to fall for my mother's feigned sincerity, so I forced a reply, wanting her to know I was doing fine without her.

"I'm doing great," I said. "Aunt Bertha treats me very well, and I'm expected to deliver in two weeks."

"What are you going to name him?"

This was "quintessential mom," who always got right down to brass tacks: *How are you? What's his name going to be?*

"Jonathan, after grandpa John." Grandpa John was the grandfather I'd visited in Shreveport when I was young. "Aunt Bertha is going to let me choose the middle name, which will be Arthur."

My mother shot back an immediate criticism.

"Why would you name him Arthur? That's not a good name. It's an old man's name."

My mother's words were like rapid machine gun fire.

I rolled my eyes and sighed. Of course Mom would think Arthur was a poor choice of names. Arthur was her first husband and Tonya's father. I'd decided on this name because he'd been there for me far more frequently than my biological father, Melvin. Birthdays, holidays, special events— Arthur was always present. What he provided for Tonya, he provided for me. He was a special man and the only real father I'd ever known. I'd had a special relationship with him, and my decision was made without regard to Arthur being one of my mother's ex-spouses.

I was irritated already, and the conversation wasn't five minutes old yet. "Mom, what do you want?"

"What are your plans for your baby?" she asked, emphasizing the word "your" in a hurtful way. She was well aware of my plan to let Aunt Bertha adopt Jonathan, and the question seemed pointless.

"Aunt Bertha is adopting the baby. You already know that."

That's when my world shifted again, tilting even farther on its axis.

"Have you thought about this, Melanie?" she asked in an exasperated tone. "What will he be to you? Will you and Aunt Bertha pretend he's your cousin? This will certainly be awkward at family reunions. Why do you feel the need to give the baby away?"

The awkwardness of future family reunions seemed to be a distant issue not worth considering. I began to cry. With two weeks until my expected date of delivery, Mom was blindsiding me. Did she want me to keep the baby so she could watch me fail miserably at childrearing while I attended college? Such a motivation seemed in keeping with my mother's personality. I couldn't fathom her reasoning, but the bottom line came down to this: After months of trying to reassure myself that I was doing the right thing, Mom was planting seeds of doubt. While it's true I'd planted seeds of my own thanks to my aunt's altered behavior, I still hadn't arrived at a definitive decision to change the existing agreement. I gave my mother the answer she surely must have already known.

"I'm doing it because I want to go to college. I want to become a doctor."

"I can help you do that. You and Jonathan can stay with me."

Something wasn't adding up. This was Mom I was talking to, the person who had declared emphatically that she didn't want to hear the pitter-patter of little feet. I wanted to believe her, but the possibility of having it all, of having a baby while I attended college, was incomprehensible. How could I trust my mother, who now, as in the past, was demonstrating erratic and contradictory behavior?

The reply was already on my tongue. "Mom, you said, and I quote, 'I have raised all the children I want to raise.' I can't believe you'd even bring this up so soon to my delivery!" I was almost yelling.

"All I'm saying is to think, Melanie. Think about what you're doing."

A few moments of silence ensued as I pondered my mother's last statement. Hadn't I thought enough? My journals were a testament to the pros and cons I had weighed and the countless hours of soul-searching I'd engaged in.

Or maybe I had indeed thought, but not clearly enough. Since leaving Reno, I'd rolled with the idea of giving the baby away, with the notion that adoption was the perfect solution. Indeed, the wording held the key: From the beginning, I was giving away *the* baby, not *my* baby.

With Mom still on the line, I silently repeated the mantra representing my entire stay in Kansas City: *I'm adopting the baby out because I am going to college.* I'd halted consideration of all other options because they didn't exist. There simply wasn't a way to do this on my own. How could a seventeen year old with a baby survive? Where would I live? Who would teach me to drive? How could I even afford a car to begin with? How could I work, go to school, and take care of a baby all at the same time? These questions, which I'd suppressed, flooded my mind because they all had only one answer: Adoption.

And then there was Aunt Bertha's feelings to consider. I'd promised her my baby, and she'd put her all into preparing for Junior. Nothing seemed crueler than taking away her dream at the last minute. True, in recent days I wasn't one hundred percent sure that adoption was the right solution given the conversation that Aunt B had had with Joyce and Joyce's children, but I was keenly aware that any change at this point would devastate my aunt. My mother was really pissing me off. Given everything she'd said and done in the past months, how could she try to jump back into the picture at the eleventh hour?

Mom broke the awkward silence. "Move back to Reno," she said bluntly. "You can live with me. If you want to go to college, that's fine. What I'm telling you, Melanie, is that I'll help you." There was no warmth in the offer, no long, persuasive argument for her change of heart. This was my mother, who was always committed to a destination, not the scenic route.

Mom had promised many things in the past, but in the end she'd always failed me. But maybe my absence and the imminent birth of Jonathan had caused her to soften. Maybe she wanted to make it up to me, realizing after five months that she *did* want me in her life. Perhaps warmth, even just a smidgeon, would emerge once she held her grandson.

Unable to know what was behind my mother's offer, I gave her an answer to end the conversation on an indefinite note.

"Okay," I said. "I'll think about it, but I gotta go."

I didn't have anything to do at that moment, but my mind was spinning, racing, twirling, doubt and hope dueling in my mind. I'd wondered on my own about the wisdom of playing incubator for Aunt B's Junior. Was my mother now offering an alternative that would release me from my agreement and allow me to keep the baby that had become so real since my second ultrasound? Could I actually make the transition from incubator to real person?

I wrote in my journal non-stop for one hour that evening, putting all of my fears and frustrations onto paper. My hand could hardly keep up with my thoughts as I speculated about the reason for Mom's phone call, as well as my renewed doubts about adoption. I wished the pages could talk back, giving me wisdom and advice, and in a sense they could. One writes in a journal in order to process thoughts and actions, hoping for both catharsis and revelation.

I paused, slipping the pen behind my hair, and stared at the wall while I rubbed my belly, my hand tracing familiar circles. But I rubbed it in a way I hadn't before, beginning with a wide circle encompassing my entire abdomen, narrowing each motion until I imagined my hand was over Jonathan's heart. I felt a kick. I closed my eyes and took a deep breath, choosing to hope that, against all odds, some bit of magic would enable me to keep my baby.

Maybe I was on the verge of a revelation after all.

* * *

A few days passed, and in the course of casual conversation, I found myself agreeing with Aunt Bertha's comments about her plans for Jonathan in the context of a mother-son relationship. But I was lying. A revelation had indeed been materializing in the past forty-eight hours, one that would send ripples through the lives of many people: If I chose to take my mother at her word—a risky proposition, to be sure—I might have it all, college and my baby. I was about to take away all of Aunt B's methodical planning for Junior, and she didn't know it.

May third was drawing close, and I knew I had to give voice to my misgivings. I wished someone else could break the news to her, just as Darryl's mother had informed my mother about the pregnancy, some third party that would jump in and say, "Melanie is keeping her baby!" But that wasn't going to happen, and in light of the many times I'd realized the necessity to be an adult, I knew the task fell to me and no one else. It would probably be the most important and difficult of all the decisions in my life thus far, but if I was about to have a baby, I had to be the grown up. Asking someone to deliver bad news was for little girls.

Be a grown up, Melanie. Be an adult. The words echoed inside my mind over and over like a mantra.

I summoned all the inward strength I had since I knew that Aunt Bertha had tremendous power over me. She was a religious person who knew that I, too, prayed. She could, if she chose, lay a heavy guilt trip on me for going back on my word and point out that I was depriving her of a lifelong dream at the last minute. This was one instance where I thought she could overcome her uncertainties in very short order with some sharp rhetoric.

I said it over dinner. "Aunt Bertha, I'm really sorry, but I don't think I can give Jonathan to you." I couldn't look her in the eye. My own eyes were fixed on my hands, which nervously tugged at each other in my lap. I started to cry.

Her initial reply was surprising. Maybe the word "think" had resonated with my aunt, causing her to realize that some degree of ambivalence was still lodged in my thinking.

"Baby," she said, "it's okay to have these thoughts. Things will be just fine for Junior and me. You know I'll take good care of him. You want to go to college, right?"

The last sentence seemed very calculated, taking direct aim at my dream of going into medicine. And yet everything she said had been correct. In fact, I knew she could do a far better job of taking care of Jonathan than I could. She was a career nurse who owned her house, and I of course wanted to go to college. I reverted to the only response I could make.

"Mom said she would help me with Jonathan and watch him while I was in school."

My aunt's tone of voice quickly switched to one of extreme exasperation as she went on the offense.

"Melanie, has your mother done anything for you while you've been living here? I'm the one who made sure you got to school, went to the doctor, ate the right foods, and took care of you while you were on bed rest. Really, Melanie, where has she been?"

I wondered if my aunt and my mother had argued recently, my mother's offer representing a way to get back at her sister for whatever had come between them. Still, Aunt B's words were harsh but valid. My mother had done nothing for me in the last five months.

"But she said she'd help me," I stammered defensively, and even I had to admit that my defense was shaky. If my mother were on trial and I was defending her, I'd lose the case, hands down. All evidence pointed to her lack of responsibility and flakiness.

Aunt Bertha's cheerful face grew sallow and dull. I was a dark moon eclipsing the sun in her life. Her sun's name was Junior.

"I'm sorry," I repeated, not knowing what else to say. I wished that my mother and my aunt could battle it out among themselves, leaving me neutral in whatever conflict might exist between them.

I went to my room, which had all of the special touches my aunt had provided: the stuffed teddy bears, the burgundy recliner, the lace curtains, and so much more. I'd never had a room so nice, nor had I ever felt so special and loved before moving to Kansas City. I picked up a teddy bear and sobbed into its soft fur. I was about to give it all away, and move back to Reno, as if my life were a board game and my "token" was a die cast Greyhound bus.

Ambivalence. My aunt had indeed chosen to exercise her power over me. Aunt B would be left with nothing, perhaps thinking that God himself had let her down. She would be left living in a void after months of hope. I wanted to keep Jonathan, but I wasn't sure what was best for *him*, and wasn't that the real question that needed to be answered? Why had my mother waited so long to advance her proposal? I was mad at her.

I heard Aunt Bertha's footsteps in the hallway.

"I'm washing my hands of this!" she said, coming through the doorway. "You're on your own. And know this: I'm not taking time off if I'm scheduled to work when the baby arrives." Her expression was a combination of anger and hurt.

Was she really going to wash her hands of the whole matter? Her remark left me feeling dirty and tainted. I had already been made to feel dirty—me, the unmarried, pregnant seventeen year old who'd been whispered about and judged by so many strangers. Now I wasn't even sincerely wanted by my aunt any longer. Yes, I was dirty. I had caused my aunt considerable pain, and I felt like someone she should rid herself of. I was residue, gum that sticks to the bottom of a sneaker and cannot easily be disposed of.

Aunt Bertha wasn't going to be there for me any longer, but I couldn't hop on a Greyhound and hightail it to Reno. My doctors were in Kansas City, plus I needed to graduate from high school. Jonathan and I would have to make it on our own somehow.

My aunt was still standing in the doorway, sensing my pain. "Yes, I am washing my hands of this," she reiterated.

My aunt's sense of power, together with the guilt she was doling out, continued to pound me like a hammer. I wasn't sure if the doctor who would deliver the baby would be Dr. Quinn. I might be alone, going through a major life experience with not a single friendly face in the large hospital.

I was clearly the bad guy, the one who hadn't kept her word, but I stopped further tears from forming. I didn't want my aunt to see my own pain or that I was allowing myself to feel sad.

The realization hit a second time: Jonathan and I would have to make it on our own.

* * *

On May sixth, I felt contractions that reminded me of menstrual cramps. They weren't frequent; they came with enough time between them for me to relax and wonder if another were going to follow. Each time, another cramp indeed bore down on my belly. I called Aunt B at work despite her previous harsh language, and she said she would be home in two hours. She was neither indifferent nor excited, just matter-of-fact.

Two hours seemed a long time to wait.

I called Labor and Delivery, the number for which was on the refrigerator. The nurse told me that the contractions were not close enough for me to come in. Rather, she suggested I take a bath. I sat in the warm water, which indeed eased the contractions. I wasn't necessarily afraid of the contractions—I knew exactly what my body was doing—but I wanted someone to be with me.

By the time Aunt Bertha arrived home, the contractions were coming faster. Still, we waited a few more hours until I pleaded to be taken to the hospital. As I waited for Aunt B to make a decision, my mind wandered to Wyandotte's senior prom, which was the following night. Having attended my junior prom with Darryl in Jackson, I didn't think I'd be missing out on much. I had more serious matters to attend to.

* * *

I was finally brought to the hospital and ushered to the triage area on the Labor and Delivery floor. The on-call physician checked my cervix and declared that it was dilated enough so that I could be admitted. The staff transferred me to a labor room and attached contraction and fetal heart-rate monitors to my abdomen. I was glad Aunt B was there, even though she didn't really want to be. The first labor nurse was friendly and tucked me in. The contractions continued, and I wondered when I would be given an epidural. I could have told them then and there that I was ready, but the nurse explained I'd have to wait until my labor was further along.

When the shift changed, Aunt Bertha went down to the cafeteria, with the next nurse chatting with a second nurse (standing on the other side of me) about the latest hospital gossip and what was happening on a soap opera they both enjoyed. I felt ignored and had no interest in what they were saying. They certainly didn't appear to be concerned about me, the large, pregnant teenager literally lying between their banter. I suspected that they regarded me as just another black teen on Medicaid, one of many they had encountered in their careers. I didn't have the courage or energy to ask them to stop talking about superficial topics and give me their attention. When my contractions picked up, however, I had to speak.

"May I have an epidural now?" I interrupted.

Distracted, the first nurse turned to me, surprised that I would dare interrupt a single precious moment from one of the many days of their lives.

"The doctor has to check you first," she replied, resuming her conversation with the other nurse.

"Do you know when he might get here?" I asked.

Her look of annoyance intensified.

"I'll go check to see if he's around," she said, upset that I was actually asking her to work.

To see if he's around. Was he down at the corner pool hall? At home? Didn't they know if he was even in the hospital?

Fortunately, Dr. Quinn was on call and emerged twenty minutes later. I was glad to see a familiar face as opposed to one of the other doctors in his group.

"Let's see where you are now," he said, placing a glove on his hand so he could check my cervix. "Five centimeters," he declared.

"May I please have a epidural?" I asked. "Pleeeeeeeze?"

He nodded, and the anesthesiologist was paged.

The epidural felt like a cool trickle down my back. I couldn't imagine having gone without this relief any longer.

When Aunt B returned from dinner, a lot had happened. It was lights, camera, action, and time to push, a performance in which the baby had the starring role. Aunt B held my hand. She'd taken a long time to eat her dinner (I suppose witnessing the delivery would be painful since it was no longer going to result in her being a mother), but she was there now, and I was thankful that a family member was next to my bed. I wanted to express my gratitude and tell her how much I needed her, but after our unpleasant exchanges, I didn't know how.

I bore down again and again, feeling terribly exposed. I had a bowel movement but didn't care. I was shaking and just wanted the baby to be out. It was another of my surreal experiences, with my mind feeling as if it were observing the whole scene from above.

"I'm going to have to make a little cut," Dr. Quinn said from behind his mask. He was referring to an episiotomy, a slight incision in the perineum made during childbirth to prevent damage to the vaginal area. At this point, I didn't care about any "cut."

"Forceps," the doctor said.

Forceps? What were those? I saw the assistant hand Dr. Quinn long metal instruments.

"I need to apply these to deliver the baby," he said.

The forceps scared me. They looked cold and clinical, like instruments of torture. I had told the anesthesiologist I didn't want to see the needle, and I should have told Dr. Quinn that I didn't want to see the forceps either. Meanwhile, everyone was telling me to push. Over and over again came the order: "Push! Push!" I felt as if I'd pushed all I could. Exhausted, I wanted to give up. Had I not won an Olympic gold medal for pushing?

"Can't you do a C-section or something?" I asked wearily.

The doctor said it was too late for that, but to please give the best push I could muster. I pushed one final time, long and hard, and he delivered the baby using the forceps, which are long, shiny instruments tantamount to a clamp to pull the baby's head through the birth canal. Someone said, "It's a boy."

After a few minutes, they placed the baby on my chest, and he felt so heavy—he weighed ten pound, ten ounces. I noticed he was pale, but I had no real emotional response yet. All I could think is that *this baby is too heavy to be on my chest right now.* I therefore asked Aunt Bertha to hold him.

"Congratulations!" Dr. Quinn said before whispering to his assistant that I had sustained a third-degree tear. Even with the episiotomy, my ten-pound son had had trouble squeezing into the world.

Jonathan had finally made his appearance, perhaps destined to be a strong, powerful man. I was proud.

I looked at Aunt Bertha while Dr. Quinn stitched me up, wondering what was going through her mind as she held my baby, the one she had labeled Junior for so many months. It must have been a bittersweet moment for her. She leaned over so I could see him. I was amazed yet again at his size. I couldn't tell at that moment who he looked like, but he was mine: Jonathan Arthur Watkins, born May 7, 1994 at 11: 29 p.m.

I was asked to complete some routine forms the next day, which was Mother's Day. One form had a line reading "Name of mother." I instinctively wrote my mother's name on the line before realizing that *I* was now the mother. I crossed out Mom's name and wrote my own.

The nurse brought Jonathan to me for his feeding, and his body felt so good in my arms, as if he were meant to be there. I knew I'd made the right decision.

Graduation was in three weeks, after which we'd be back on our way to Reno. I was going to give my mother a chance, for better or worse. My Aunt B generously paid for one-way airline tickets for my son and me. I thought it showed a lot of love, forgiveness, and character on my aunt's part.

Most importantly, however, I wasn't traveling alone this time. I was with Jonathan. The time of decision-making was over. It had been a long road from Jackson to Kansas City, with the events in between seeming like those from an odyssey one reads about in classic poetry. In the long run, however, my struggles had paid off. I had made my choice, and the baby was mine.

That didn't mean I wasn't afraid of what lay ahead. The true odyssey was just beginning.

* * *

11

The University of Nevada is a beautiful campus, with trees, a lake, and modern buildings like most other colleges. Ironically, it's located in downtown Reno, near casinos where the youngest college students can't drink, gamble, or even work. But it was the college that I'd chosen—I had no regrets simply because of its odd juxtaposition to Nevada's financial life blood—and I was very excited about beginning the Howard Hughes summer program, which provided housing on campus, classes in math and science, and even the opportunity to tutor these subjects. The idea of tutoring increased my anxiety but I believed that it would make for an interesting transition into my new world. I couldn't help but wonder if I was up to the task given that I'd been to five different high schools, one of them twice—I was in the Health Sciences program with an emphasis on pre-med—but I had confidence in my abilities.

My new world. It was again surreal, but despite some butterflies in my stomach—to be expected—the complete repainting of the landscape of my life was welcome this time around. I'd had Jonathan and was attending college. To paraphrase the psalm, I had indeed walked through the valley of the shadow of death, but I had made it through thanks to many good people, and, I believe, God, the very God Grandpa John had told me about so many distant summers ago. I had some scars, figuratively and literally, but that was okay. I was on the right path for a change.

* * *

When I arrived in Reno, baby in tow, I was happy to see Arthur at the airport, he and his wife Linda standing not far away from my mother.

Arthur and Linda had driven up from Los Angeles and purchased and crib and playpen for Jonathan. I was overjoyed to be there, and having Arthur greet me made it all the more special. His generosity had not changed through the years.

Jonathan was only three weeks old, but the Howard Hughes Medical Institute program was starting in only two—you play the hand you're dealt—so it was time to get into gear and start yet another new phase of my life. I had performed under pressure before, and I could do it again, but I was still nervous

My dormitory roommate was Sarah, a student from Reno who wanted to become a marine biologist. She was nineteen, and I liked her from the first day I met her. She was a portrait of the Midwest, her hair long, with the top pulled straight back over her head. She was down-to-earth, smart, and focused. There were many other women in the program—most in their late twenties—who seemed to be very confident and strong. Many said they were envious of me for starting my academic journey right out of high school. Little did they know the price I had paid to do so.

I didn't tell anyone I had a baby for the first week of the program. I was conditioned for fear after many months of feeling that a bright, garish spotlight was shining on me, the promiscuous teen, and I thought students might judge me for being an unwed teenage mother, wondering why I was even there. Didn't people such as me work at 7-Eleven or Target? At seventeen, I thought the administration itself might ask me to leave the program if it was aware I had a baby. I therefore kept Jonathan a secret, as much as it pained me.

On most weekends (and during a few evenings a week), I left the dorm, taking the bus so I could see Jonathan. I lied to Sarah on these occasions, telling her that my mother was ill and that I had to periodically check on her health. I dared not tell Sarah the truth since I felt a tremendous amount of shame for being a young mother. By the same token, I was ashamed of *being* ashamed—ashamed for having Jonathan. I wanted to be proud of being a mother, even at seventeen, but I wasn't willing to risk putting myself in a position I couldn't explain or defend. I didn't think I had the "feel" for college yet or its unique rhythms.

The administrators of the program were Ms. King, Dr. Gubanich, and Dr. Mead. Doctors Gubanich and Mead were professors of science at UNR, and Ms. King was director of the tutoring program on campus. (The Howard Hughes Medical Institute or "HHMI" was essentially operating as a consortium with the University of Nevada, Reno.) I admired and respected each one of these people, who were genuine, kind, and committed to their students' greatness. Ms. King was known for giving great pep talks and validating the students she worked with—her "Hughesians". Doctors Gubanich and Mead expected more than we expected from ourselves. They gave us what I had always wanted and needed (and what I felt some of the teachers at Callaway never could provide): They pushed us and challenged us to be out very best. I must have always exhibited an exuberance and lifelong desire for learning and advancement, for they recognized a spark in me and kindled it with their unending enthusiasm. I worked hard and gave the program my all.

I was in my dorm room with Sarah a few weeks into the program. As we were getting ready for bed, we started chatting idly about what college life would be like in the fall. Sarah said it would be great fun, with numerous opportunities, such as parties, joining sororities, ordering pizza at midnight, and even late-night study groups. It all sounded intriguing, but I couldn't allow myself the luxury of getting excited about such activities for the simple reason that I knew I could never participate in them. Mom had made it very clear upon my arrival in Reno that she would take care of Jonathan, but not to the extent that I would be free to socialize. I could hear her voice in my mind. *This is your child, Melanie. Yes, I'm helping, but I'm not the full-time mother. I'm not watching Jonathan while you party.* I stared at the ceiling and tried to stifle my tears.

"What's wrong, Melanie?" Sarah asked.

"I won't be able to do all those things," I answered. I paused, trying to force the words out. "I have a baby."

"What?" Sarah asked in a tone of disbelief.

"I had a son seven weeks ago. My mother takes care of him for me so I can participate in the Hughes program. I haven't told anyone because I don't want to be judged or kicked out of the program." I wiped away my tears with the sleeve of my nightgown.

Sarah's response was surprisingly supportive.

"They can't kick you out for having a baby!" she said. "In fact, they would probably want to help you."

"How?" I asked. I was shocked at my roommate's suggestion.

"Well, maybe you can get additional financial aid or something," Sarah said with a note of encouragement. "I think you should absolutely tell Miss King." Not only had Sarah not been judgmental, but she thought that the situation might actually work in my favor. I wasn't so sure, however.

"I can't. I'd be too embarrassed. She currently thinks a lot of me, and I wouldn't want to let her down by telling her I was a teen mother."

The feeling of shame washed over me again as I lay in bed. I had deceived everyone in the program, students and professors alike. Tonya had told me that if I were woman enough to sleep with a man and have his baby, I should be woman enough to accept the consequences, but that was easier said than done. The consequences thus far had been burdensome and difficult. Even professionals—adult counselors and social workers—had looked at me with stern eyes, their voices disparaging. Consequently, I was still struggling with my identity as a seventeen-year-old mother.

The next day, I focused on continuing to excel in the program. The HHMI classes were ending in a few weeks, and there was to be a party to celebrate our achievements. I struggled over whether or not to bring Jonathan. I figured I didn't have anything to lose at this point since the administration couldn't kick me out of the program now. More importantly, I didn't want to be ashamed anymore. Hiding a baby was more of a fictional comedy for Hollywood, and my life had been fodder for drama, not laughs. I was finished with shame even though I might feel uncomfortable as a teen mother at times. I was going to write a different script.

I took the bus home, transferring downtown to another bus that stopped in front of my apartment complex, so there wasn't any real walking involved—just a few steps. At times, it seemed that my life revolved around bus schedules. I couldn't go to certain suburban areas because the bus routes didn't include them. I was further limited because the frequency with which the buses ran varied depending on the time of day, or the day of the week. Sometimes, the buses ran every twenty minutes. Other times, they ran every hour, and missing an hourly bus was devastating. Not only was the wait at the stop maddening, but I'd have to explain to people at my destination, such as a doctor's receptionist, why I was late, pleading with her to still fit me into the schedule since I couldn't imagine having to go through the same ordeal all over again.

* * *

The party was scheduled for 3 p.m. on a Saturday, which was better than Sunday, when the busses run hourly. My mother said she had "commitments," so I couldn't ask her for a ride. I didn't know how to drive yet, so borrowing the car wasn't an option, nor did I want to ask any of the students for a lift since I felt it was my responsibility to arrange my own transportation. It might have been because I hadn't introduced them to Jonathan yet, or perhaps I wanted to see if I could get there by myself, even though it would be a challenging bus ride. I wanted to know that I had what it took to be a mother in all circumstances. I was just starting on the odyssey of motherhood, and I would face far greater challenges in the future.

Mom was waiting for me when I arrived home to pick up Jonathan. I thanked her for watching him—she was beginning to soften little by little to having a baby in the house—and I picked up my son from his crib. He looked especially cute in his light blue outfit, and I grabbed his baby bag and made sure it was filled with all of the necessities a new parent must tote everywhere the baby goes: diapers, wipes, bottles with formula, and pacifier. The fold-up stroller was leaning against the wall next to the front door, so I grabbed it for the short walk to the bus stop. Both of my hands were full, but I made it to the stop just in time for the next bus.

As the bus lurched away from the curb, I clumsily made my way to a seat in the front, an area usually reserved for the elderly or the disabled. I sat next to a woman in her late sixties who looked at me disapprovingly. I certainly felt a bit "disabled" myself at the moment, and I wondered if her glaring look was because I was a very young mother or because I was laden with so many things—baby, stroller, and bag. I kept an eye out since I would have gladly relinquished my seat if an elderly or disabled person needed my seat, but at that moment, I needed to collapse. My arms were already tired. I was excited that the other students were going to meet Jonathan, but I was also nervous. Pride and fear drifted in and out of my thoughts—this emotional cocktail was nothing new—but I knew that bringing him along was yet another important step in my assuming the role of grown-up.

As if on cue, Jonathan started screaming (or at least it sounded like screaming even though it was only loud crying). I was trapped on a moving bus with a two-month-old who was unhappy about something, and I wasn't at all sure what that "something" was.

I checked his diaper. Not wet.

I gave him his bottle. Not hungry.

I rocked him gently. Not effective.

I started sweating. Was the driver going to kick me off the bus?

"You can train your child, or your child can train you," the cranky old lady snickered. She sounded like an older version of Joyce's daughter Erika. The comment had been a cheap shot. I guess she expected me to be an abusive mother and slap my child into silence.

I rolled my eyes, trying to keep from being disrespectful, but the elderly woman saw that I was struggling. Her demeanor made me feel even more incompetent. Would I know what to do if I were thirty or forty? (Would the woman even dare have made such a comment if I were older?) Would Jonathan be crying if his father were present—or *anyone* familiar? I had no one to ask for advice and wondered why Mom couldn't have taken just a few minutes to give me a ride. Even though she was doing a good job, she wasn't cutting me much slack, as if she wanted me to wear a scarlet A on my chest as a reminder of my past. But that is who my mother was. Love always seemed conditional in some, way, shape, or form.

Jonathan kept crying, and at seventeen, I didn't have the guts to stand up for myself. Ignoring the stinging comment from the old woman, I was still reminded of how out of control I felt.

We neared the downtown transfer station. Jonathan was still crying, although he'd thankfully brought his wails down a few decibels. Placing him in his stroller, I pushed him around for fifteen minutes, and he quieted down before falling fast asleep. That was all it had been! He was cranky because he was tired!

When the next bus arrived, I gently lifted him from the stroller, careful not to wake him, and placed him on my shoulder. I deftly folded up the stroller with one arm—I was becoming a pro at juggling my baby accoutrements—got on the bus, and made my way to the back, where there were less people. I sank down into a seat and rocked both of us. I knew we were going to make it to UNR on time and felt a wave of relief—and accomplishment.

When we got off at the university stop, Jonathan was miraculously asleep. I walked to the dorm, where the party was being held in the ground floor lobby, glad to see everyone. Walking over to me with a smile, Ms. King unburdened my arms of the baby bag and stroller, leaning them against the wall.

"Who is this little one?" she asked. "Is this your brother?"

I smiled nervously. It was the moment of truth. "This is Jonathan. He's my son."

Every student within earshot turned towards us immediately. I braced myself, unsure of what their reaction was going to be.

"Melanie," said Ms. King, "you have a son! Why didn't you tell us?" She was smiling with disbelief.

I replied with a boldface lie in order to avoid a direct answer to her question.

"Well, Mom helps me out a lot," I said. "I go home on evenings a lot and on the weekends. It wasn't too difficult."

It had been *extremely* difficult, and the past weeks represented only the first yards of a difficult road I was now traveling. But to answer Ms. King's "why" question—no, that would have entailed admitting my shame, fear, guilt, and embarrassment, and I wanted to appear strong in front of everyone.

As time wore on that day, it was a relief to see everyone getting to know my son. I could finally admit them into this part of my life. Ms. King even held Jonathan and gave him a bottle shortly after he awakened from his nap. She was like a surrogate mother, understanding and empathetic. Why hadn't I told her? I was almost certain she would have accepted me, but she and the other faculty members were the exceptions and not the rule. I had experienced harsh judgment from too many people on the long road to giving birth, including those in my own family.

The party had been a ray of sunshine. I was again reminded that there were wonderful people in the world who would not condemn me. I'm almost sure one of my Grandpa's stories in Shreveport had been on that very subject.

* * *

12

Three weeks to go and then I'm in the academic big leagues for real: college. Taking care of Jonathan for a full week gave me to time to think. (Maybe I'd been thinking *too* much, but I'd always been a reflective person, which is why I couldn't live without my journals.) I felt overwhelmed while Mom was at work. This was far different from popping over on weekends and evenings while living on the UNR campus during the summer. I was extremely tired on most days since Jonathan rarely slept through the night. How could I do this alone? Mom was certainly available . . . although she didn't go out of her way to make the time to take up the slack in caring for Jonathan. She often tried to tell me how to handle him, but she was like a stern coach shouting in plays from the sideline. Otherwise, it wasn't a team approach. What I really needed was some hands-on help. Why had my mother called me at Aunt Bertha's, urging me to return to Reno, if this was the "help" she was offering. Why had she herself demanded that I *think, think, think* about my decision to adopt? I'd envisioned quite a bit more help than I was receiving.

I was also stressed about financial aid, or the lack thereof. The University of Nevada had given me scholarships, but they barely covered the cost of tuition, books, or living expenses. Mom helped me get public assistance, but negotiating the system in Reno proved even more challenging than in Jackson. I'd also received a $2,500 stipend during the HHMI summer program, but money goes fast when there's a hungry mouth to feed at all hours of the day, plus I couldn't skimp on wipes, diapers, or clothing. I considered using a babysitter or campus childcare, but that, too, meant additional money leaving the coffer in our home. At least Jonathan qualified for WIC, a federal program for women, infants, and children that provided milk, cereal, cheese, and juice. Still, our budget was tight.

Feeling confused and adrift with the start of school bearing down on me so quickly, my thoughts gravitated to Darryl. I'd always been concerned about Jonathan not having a father in his life. Had he changed? If he could see his son and learn what I'd been through, would he finally value me and show me the love and respect I deserved? If Darryl *had* changed, then we could be a regular family, representing the best of all possible worlds. If he *hadn't* changed, maybe a baby would help him to mellow out, motivating him to meet his responsibilities. Then again, maybe he had moved, from Jackson, gotten a girlfriend, or both. Out of sight, out of mind, as the old saying goes, and Darryl had never even seen his son. Either way, I didn't think I could stay with Mom indefinitely. Once the semester began, things were going to get busier, and her rules about childcare were going to remain stringent. I knew she loved Jonathan, but her enthusiasm didn't fill the gap between what needed to be done and what she was willing to do.

I was overwhelmed. I bought a phone card and decided to contact Darryl. I had to find out where matters stood in Jackson. It was time to let Darryl know he had a son, even if nothing came of it.

"Darryl? Hi. This is Melanie."

His response was matter-of-fact, cold. The charm he occasionally showed me when I lived in Jackson wasn't coming through the telephone line. Perhaps, I thought, he was too proud (or hurt) to display emotion to the girl who'd left him. Or maybe it was gone for good.

"Yeah," he said. "Long time, no talk. You gave our baby away?"

The remark seemed as callous as when his mother had told me, "You better hope you lose that baby." Maybe he would warm up a bit if I explained how things had played out.

"No, Darryl. I decided to keep him. We're in Reno now, and he's with me at this very moment. He's so cute, Darryl! His name is Jonathan." I wanted Darryl to feel my enthusiasm.

"Oh yeah? Really? Does he look like me?"

I looked down at Jonathan. "He sure does. He has your nose." I couldn't suppress a smile as I said that. The very comment seemed to imply "family."

"You decided to keep him," Darryl said flatly. "I told you it didn't make no sense for you to give him away like that. You with Dorothy?"

It was interesting that he segued to the subject of my mother so quickly.

"Mom's helping me out, but it's hard. She's strict, and her rules are difficult to follow. I sometimes feel like Jonathan is my brother rather than my son. I'm supposed to start college in a few weeks, and money-wise, things are really tight."

Darryl didn't hesitate.

"I can help you out. I got a new job down here at the shop. It pays good money. Why you there in Nevada then? If you were down here, we could get a place and be a family." Everyone wanted to help me out—Darryl, Aunt Bertha, Tonya, Mom—and yet they had all failed me in one way or the other.

But Darryl's words were powerful. *Be a family.* Moving to Jackson might solve all my problems. I would have help with Jonathan, and hopefully Tougaloo's offer was still open.

"Darryl, let me call you back. I have to make a few other calls to see if I can do this."

I hung up and looked in my notebook for the number of the Admissions Office of Tougaloo. What if the "all expenses paid" offer had already expired? Tougaloo's week-long orientation was due to begin the following Monday, so there were only four days to settle the matter one way or the other. I was cutting things razor close, but if there was a chance I could still be admitted to the college, I wanted to know as soon as possible.

I called both the Admissions Office and the Financial Aid Office, and the staff was happy to hear of my interest in their college. I was informed that Tougaloo offered free tuition, dormitory housing, meals, books—everything. I could hardly believe my good fortune. I was eager to share my thoughts with Mom when she came home.

"Mom, I think I should go back to Jackson," I said, trying to get the words out quickly before she could pre-empt me with negativity and nay-saying. "Tougaloo is offering me a lot more financial support than UNR, and many of their pre-med students get into medical school. I think maybe I should go there instead. If I can go to college for free and then get into med school, assuming I study hard, how can I pass that up?"

Mom reached out to take Jonathan from me, as if the gesture itself was her answer. "So what does Darryl think about this?" she asked skeptically.

"Darryl has nothing to do with this. I'm only thinking about what is best for my career."

Mom wasn't buying into my argument.

"I don't know why you would want to go back down there," she said with a frustrated sigh. "You really should think about getting your associate's degree in nursing and be done with all this as quickly as possible. You don't need to be putting your son through all of these changes. You're only seventeen, Melanie, and Jon deserves to have a life that's not constantly disrupted."

On the one hand, Mom's response was logical inasmuch as Aunt B was a nurse and had done all right for herself. Also, on the surface, her answer was eminently logical. Moving children around is not an ideal option if it can be avoided, but nothing in my life in the past two years had been logical or ideal if examined from a purely rational viewpoint.

But my mother's response ultimately didn't hold any water since her otherwise sound logic was full of contradictions. I'd attended five different high schools, one of them twice, in a four-year period. I'd lived in Phoenix, Jackson, Reno and Kansas City from 1990 to 1994. How could she possibly preach to me regarding stability and raising children? My life had been disrupted many times by moves, and Mom had had a hand in all of them.

Or was there another motive behind her reluctance to have me explore the possibility of going to Tougaloo? For someone who had said she wasn't keen on having an infant around, she was happy to hold Jonathan when she came home from work each day. For all of her reticence and tough love in teaching me about the rigors of being a single mother, she seemed to want a piece of the action after all. Being a grandmother seemed to suit her . . . when she made the time for assuming the role. Indeed, she was holding my son at that very moment as if to protect him from what she believed to be my crazy schemes.

"I don't want to be a nurse," I responded. "You know my heart is set on being a doctor. This is important to me, Mom. Tougaloo is going to support me and can help make my career dreams come true. Jonathan and I are going to leave tomorrow. I already called Tougaloo, and they want to see me there on Monday."

"What?" Mom was nonplussed. "Where are you going to stay? The college isn't going to allow you to have a baby in the dormitory," she said as she bounced Jonathan on her shoulder.

She was right—and *knew* she was right. There was no family housing available on the Tougaloo campus. As always, however, I was willing to do whatever needed to be done to achieve my goals, even if I didn't have all of the details worked out.

"We might have to stay with Darryl for a bit," I admitted. "I'm not entirely sure, but I'll figure it out. I have to leave tomorrow, though, because orientation is on Monday."

My mother looked at me as if I'd lost my mind.

"With Darryl? No, you're not taking Jonathan down there," she said emphatically. "He's just three months old, and you want to subject him to a three-day bus ride? No. If this is your decision, then go to Tougaloo, but I'll take care of Jonathan until you get settled in and decide whatever it is you're going to do. You can return and get him when you have worked things out a little more carefully, but you're not going to put this baby through all of this."

She looked at Jonathan and kissed him. I would have not been surprised if she'd said, "You won't put *my* baby through all of this."

I had to take stock of my decision, if only for a moment. Was my mother right? Would I be a bad mother to take Jon on such a long trip, especially on the bus? And was I foolish to try having a relationship with Darryl again? The latter part of Mom's statement made sense, and while it was hard to imagine myself apart from my son, part of me was relieved. Reversing course so quickly and beginning college at Tougaloo would be difficult, maybe even grueling. Besides, Darryl worked during the day, and there was simply no way I was going to allow his mother to look after Jonathan. When she had expressed the hope that I would lose the baby, she lost the possibility of ever having a relationship with her grandson. It just wasn't going to happen.

"Okay, I'll go without him," I told my mother reluctantly.

It was very hard to admit to myself that I couldn't do it all, have it all, be it all. I wasn't Wonder Woman. I was a struggling teenage mother, but at the same time I was highly motivated to prove myself. I was also eager to prove to my mother as well that I could, difficulties notwithstanding, establish myself in Jackson and do whatever it took to take care of Jonathan and get my education.

Mom promised to take care of Jonathan while I was gone and drove me to the Greyhound station at 6:30 the following morning. I kissed him on the cheek, squeezed him tightly, and said, "I love you, Jonathan."

I sat, as usual, in the seat directly behind the driver to buffer myself from the louder passengers in the back, as well as the odors from the on-board restroom.

And then I cried.

What was I doing? I hadn't said a single word about my sudden change of plans to the exemplary staff at Howard Hughes or to any of my friends. I didn't think they would understand my predicament, but I nevertheless felt guilty for having to conduct my life as if I were a CIA agent. The sad reality, however, was that few people understood what it was like to be a teenage mother. In the long run, if other people judged me as being selfish or a bad mother, then so be it. I still had to pursue the two most important goals of my life: taking care of Jonathan and becoming a doctor.

The bus ride, like so many others, was long and tedious, with the desert and brown sage of Texas rolling by the window for over a day. When "The Dog" finally pulled into its exhaust-filled berth at the station, Darryl walked up and tried to give me a deep, full kiss, not a peck on the cheek. After all the time that had elapsed, the gesture felt foreign and undesirable to me, but I allowed him to do it and kissed him back. It was okay, I thought, to let him want me.

He retrieved my bags and walked me to his automobile. After a short drive, we arrived at his home, which hadn't changed at all, as if it had been frozen in time. His mother was locked in her room, watching television. And there was still the picture of Jesus hanging above Darryl's bed, and as we had sex that night, the image of Christ looking down at us was still hard for me to look at, but I'd had no boyfriends at all since leaving Darryl. I'd gained a lot of weight during my pregnancy and longed for affection and a physical connection. And wasn't Darryl the man I wanted to help establish my family, shouldering the duties of becoming an active, involved father.

* * *

I felt a surge of adrenaline the next morning. Darryl drove me to Tougaloo with the sun still low in the sky, and as I entered the campus, I felt on top of the world. He dropped me off at the Admissions Office, and I walked past the welcome sign and proceeded to the section of the building for new students with last names beginning with T through Z. I went to the appropriate desk, where a woman said, "Name?"

"Melanie Watkins," I said.

She looked through a box filled with cards, not bothering to look up or make eye contact. Didn't she realize that I was a nervous freshman and that this was my first day of college? Couldn't she have mustered enough energy for a smile?

"Here," she said in a monotone voice. "This is your class schedule. You need to go to the financial aid office, the housing office, and the cafeteria. Here's a map. You'll pick up your dorm assignment, your key, financial aid information, and your meal tickets."

It was all just routine for her.

"Thank you!" I said, hoping that my enthusiasm would be reflected back to me. She looked past me, a drone who felt no need to at least provide some encouragement during the intimidating ordeal of registration.

"Next!" she screeched.

I endured the long lines at each and every building. When I got to the dorm, it looked eerily empty. As I sat on the bare mattress, I heard a key turn in the lock. It was my roommate. The ensuing conversation was a bit of a letdown.

"Hi. I'm Tina."

"Hi. I'm Melanie Watkins."

"Where are you from?" she asked.

"Reno."

"Reno? Where's that?"

"Nevada."

"Like, um, Vegas?"

"Sure. Like Vegas."

I was frustrated that no one seemed to know that there were other cities in Nevada besides Las Vegas, but I recalled that I myself didn't know where Reno was until I'd moved there with Mom the year before. Perhaps I was fatigued.

"I'm from Jackson," she said. "I went to Murrah. What's your major?"

"Pre-med."

It felt awkward to say these words—lofty ones indeed—which would have to be earned, not just stated. The major would require long hours of hard work, the magnitude of which I couldn't yet imagine. I also felt a bit hesitant about divulging my plans to a student from the "classy" high school on the other side of town. I wondered if she was smarter than I, having had access to a consistent four-year education with some of the finer things a high school had to offer.

But I'd beaten the odds many times before. In a real sense, I'd majored in Hard Work for two years. If I could stabilize my life with Jonathan, I knew I was up to the task.

* * *

13

A new chapter was about to begin in my life, but it wasn't the chapter that I expected.

The next day was the second day of orientation, with classes beginning the day after that. I was totally ready to start my academic journey after the annoying aspects of registration were finished, but I received an unexpected call from my mother early on the morning before the first session was to begin. I was immediately worried that something had happened to Jonathan.

"Melanie, Ms. King called to ask about you and would like you to call her. She was wondering why you weren't at the Howard Hughes reception."

There had been a reception for students who'd participated in the Hughes' summer program. It was intended to help us reconnect before the beginning of the fall semester.

"I forgot to call them," I said. This was another lie. I hadn't told particpants in the Hughes program that I was heading to Jackson because I didn't want anyone to talk me out of my present plans. They wouldn't understand, and indeed, I myself didn't fully understand what was going on in my life or the choices I was making.

"She wants you to call her right away. I told her you were in Jackson, and she left her office and personal number."

Was I in trouble, or had I failed to meet some obligation for the Hughes grant? Would I have to return the stipend? Was Ms. King simply upset upset that I'd just disappeared without even a goodbye to one of my most trusted mentors? It wasn't hard to imagine that she was disappointed in a student to whom she'd given so much time and encouragement.

"Okay, Mom. I'll give her a call."

Checking my clock, I saw that it was 6:30 PST. After lunch, I went straight from the dining hall to a payphone. I glanced at the phone number Mom had jotted down on a piece of scratch paper, then dialed it.

"Hi, Ms. King. This is Melanie. I'm sorry to have called so early in the morning, but—"

"Melanie!" she interrupted me. "I'm so glad you called. What are you doing in Jackson?"

It was a difficult question to answer in light of the fact that Ms. King had been so nurturing to me thus far. She was a large woman with a thick Boston accent, and she always had confidence when it came to tackling tough problems. Her office walls and shelves were filled with plaques, posters, and collectibles from all over the world, many saying something positive or affirming. She was a warm, maternal figure—more so than my own mother—and she deserved an honest response. I therefore told her about my financial concerns, explaining that Tougaloo appeared to be "a sure thing." I wouldn't have to pay anything, and the college graduated a higher degree of black pre-med students than any other school in Mississippi.

"Where do you really want to be, Melanie? If you had enough money, would you still be at UNR?" He voice was honest, challenging. She could sense my indecision.

"Well, UNR, of course."

I was eager to start chemistry and biology classes with many of the other Hughes students. We'd relied on each other during the summer, and I knew I could count on them for friendship and academic support. And the Hughes' staff, of course, was a resource that would be invaluable as I started the regular semester.

"But I'm already here," I said with regret. Had I burned an important bridge to my future?

Ms. King was undeterred. "Melanie, we have money for you. I spoke with Doctor Mead and Doctor Gubanich, and we made some calls to the

Financial Aid Department. We have a terrific work-study program, and you can even work in my office. There's enough money to cover your first year."

I was once more overwhelmed, as if I had won the Lottery, but there were still formidable obstacles to returning to Reno.

"I don't have any money to return," I told her. "Not even enough for bus fare. Even if I did, I'd miss the first day of classes. I don't know what to do."

Her response was to the point. "We'll fly you back."

"Thank you, Ms. King, but I could never pay you back. I—"

"That's not a problem, Melanie. We've already made airline reservations for you. The flight leaves Jackson tomorrow at 6 a.m."

My mind was spinning like an out-of-control carnival ride. I was grateful that Ms. King and the others would do this for me, but I was scared. Was there really enough money? Every time I thought I could squeeze by financially, the money was never what I anticipated. And what about Darryl? How would he react? Would he let me leave? Worse, would he follow me and harm me for misleading him? And what was in store as far as living with Mom if I returned to Reno? How would we negotiate the parenting duties since she was so domineering on some points? Last of all, what about Tougaloo? I'd already enrolled and eaten in their dining hall. Would I have to pay them for my registration and brief stay? Weighing the pros and cons was a task more suited for someone with the wisdom of Solomon. I was just a single mom trying to "get by."

"Just go to the registration office," Ms. King said. "Tell them that you've changed your mind, see what they have to say, and then call me back."

To stay or not to stay: that was the question. But there was no time for deliberation. The decision had to be made quickly.

"Wow," I said into the phone receiver. "I've already started orientation down here, and—"

"The plane ticket is waiting for you, Melanie," said Ms. King, almost unwilling to take "no" for an answer.

I thanked her and did as she asked. It was great that the people at UNR wanted me back so badly, but the people at Tougaloo's Admissions Office weren't especially happy about my change of heart. I would have some minor fees to sort out, but they were not going to make me liable for the tuition.

And yet I had no one to discuss this with because everyone always had their own opinions about what was best for me. My gut instinct was that UNR would be a better bet since I'd been comfortable with the very supportive Hughes' staff, plus they'd gone out of their way to show how much they cared about me. In Jackson, my only connection was with Darryl, and that was a relationship that had many unknown variables. Maybe it would be best to leave that equation unsolved. As for Tougaloo, the summer program I'd attended there had been brief and hadn't resulted in my making many friends. I decided to call Mom since Ms. King had contacted her directly. I was naturally uncomfortable asking my mother for advice—my mom, who often had a self-centered agenda for her actions, but I had to run this by someone, and at least Mom had bothered to relay Mrs. King's message. That counted for an awful lot.

"Mom," I began, "Ms. King said that UNR found financial aid for me and that they'll fly me back to Reno. What do you think about her idea?"

"My hands are full, Melanie, but if they have financial aid for you, then fine. I took a week off from work, but I'm returning soon, and Jonathan will need childcare."

She hadn't answered my question as much as outlined her own obligations and limitations, but I shouldn't have expected otherwise.

I missed Jonathan very much, and Mom's remark, coupled with the incentives Miss King was offering, helped seal the deal in my mind. The issue of who would take care of Jonathan in Jackson was still nebulous. I would therefore return to Reno. I called Miss King and told her that I appreciated everything she had done and would be returning the next day.

That left Darryl. Literally.

"Hi, Darryl," I began. "I was talking to some people from UNR. They now have financial aid for me and want me to fly back to start classes there."

I waited anxiously for his reply.

"Melanie, you need to be right here. With me. You don't know what you want. You keep listenin' to everybody else."

There was an element of truth in his comment, but I was returning to UNR. My mind was made up.

"But this is a great opportunity for me," I said, "and I really miss Jonathan." Without really thinking carefully about my next words, I said, "And maybe you could join us in Reno."

There was an ominous silence on the other end of the line. I had clearly caught him off guard, but I didn't know whether he'd be pleased or angry at my suggestion.

"I've got a job *here*. I don't know nuthin 'bout no Reno."

"Well, you know *me*. And you love me and want to see Jonathan, right?"

Darryl had only seen photos of his son, and I thought that Jonathan might be the best trump card to play to see if Darryl really wanted to entertain moving.

"Darryl?"

"Yeah?"

"Mechanics are needed everywhere. You could make good money in Reno. And like you said, we could be a family."

It occurred to me even as I was speaking that I was trying to convince myself as much as Darryl about the feasibility of the plan. I'd been in Jackson less than thirty-six hours and hadn't really gotten to know Darryl again. Was he still drinking? Did he still suffer from mood swings? My invitation represented a big gamble, but I couldn't count on my mother for anything except part-time help, and my plan to attend Tougaloo had been predicated, in part, on finding out whether it was possible to give Jonathan a father, plus provide the help I myself needed.

"All right," Darryl said at last. "I'm gonna come up there for you. We can be a family." He paused. "You sure you wanna do this?"

"I'm sure."

"When you leavin'? You want me to take you to the bus station?"

"No, not the bus station. The airport."

Darryl agreed.

I felt that my situation was changing. I'd be starting my studies as a pre-med student in Reno, and I'd return there by plane, not bus. And with any luck, Jonathan, Darryl, and I might become a family. It would be awkward at first, but maybe we would grow into it.

Maybe.

Darryl and I said our goodbyes the next day at the airport. I really didn't know if I would ever see him again because I was not at all sure that he was serious about moving to Reno. If he came, maybe things would be better since we would both be away from Jackson. He'd had to toe the line in the military, and by analogy, maybe a change in environment would give him a fresh outlook on life. And if he asked me, I would be his wife.

* * *

Mom met me at the airport with Jonathan. The past few days had been a whirlwind of confusion about school and family, and I could barely catch my breath as I saw my mother and son waiting for me. I hugged and kissed Jonathan over and over and was surprised that I had missed him so much after so short a period of time.

School was now starting, and although I didn't feel ready for classes—a vacation from all of the recent melodrama would have been nice—I knew that I alone had made the decision to return to Reno despite input from Ms. King, Mom, and Darryl. I would now have to live up to my own expectations.

I called Sarah, who was excited that I was back in town, and we planned to meet at the bookstore. Meanwhile, I had to pick up orientation information, stop by the Financial Aid Office, and then head to the bookstore. After my experiences in Jackson only two days earlier, it was a classic case of "déjà vu all over again." Fortunately (and not surprisingly), Ms. King helped out, making the arduous process of registration as smooth as possible.

The bookstore was packed with students looking for their texts, pens, highlighters, and notebooks. Spotting Sarah, I walked up behind her and put my hands in front of her eyes. "Guess which pre-med student is start-ing at UNR today?" I asked.

"Melanie!" she cried, whirling around.

I was euphoric as we hugged—and happy that I hadn't missed my classes despite my two about-turns during the past week. I was happy to be near Jonathan again, as well as happy about embarking on my dream of becoming a doctor. I'd come a long way from Callaway High and the Discovery Clinic.

I registered for twelve credits: Math, Chemistry, and English. Sarah and I were both taking Chemistry 101 with Dr. LeMay, an older, bald-ing man with white hair, glasses, and a warm, open smile. He wasn't the intimidating college teacher I expected to meet, the kind who walks into class, immediately starts teaching, and asks as many esoteric questions as possible in order to make students feel uncomfortable. Indeed, he told a couple of jokes to lighten up the atmosphere as soon as possible. "Henry was a chemist," Dr. LeMay said, "but he isn't anymore. He got H20 mixed up with H2S04, the latter being sulfuric acid. Poor Henry. Thirst can be a dangerous thing."

The class chuckled, surprised by our professor's joke, even if it didn't produce belly laughs. But Dr. LeMay wasn't finished with his stand-up comedy yet.

"Two peanuts were walking side by side late one night," he said. "No other peanuts were around, so it was a shame when one of them was assaulted."

The joke was corny, as was the first, but it helped ease tension among the freshmen.

As I looked down the rows of the large lecture hall, it was apparent that students in the front row exhibited a more serious demeanor. They seemed intense and asked more questions. I felt jealous of their boldness and confi-dence. Although college seemed more manageable than I'd thought thanks to Dr. LeMay's disarming humor, I also realized that that there would be a great deal more responsibility over the next four years than any I'd been given in high school or my summer programs on college campuses. There would be no reminders of when assignments were due, no one looking over my shoulder to see if I was taking good notes. I'd have to stay on top of things, but all in all, I was invigorated. I wanted to be at UNR—and for all four years.

* * *

My classes finished at 3 p.m. that day, and I wanted to stop by the baby-sitter that Mom had recommended by way of a contact she had at work. (Mom was still employed by Uncle Sam.) Holding Jonathan, Mom met me at in the parking lot and then rushed to an appointment on the other side of town. Not surprisingly, she didn't have time to take me to the woman's home. I was therefore relieved to learn that the babysitter's house was only a block from the bus stop as Jonathan and I stepped down to the curb. See-ing a torn screen door ahead, I checked the scratch paper to make sure I had the right address for Mrs. Cager, the woman who would ostensibly be tak-ing care of my son. I was at the right house, but I wondered how effective a torn screen door would be at preventing a small child from finding its way to the street (even though Jonathan was too young to even crawl yet). The front door was wide open.

I walked up to the house and saw a woman in her seventies watching TV.

"Come on in, baby," she said nonchalantly, hardly taking her eye from the screen.

"Are you Ms. Cager?" I asked,

She sat on a faded sofa, a wood-framed antique mirror hanging just above it. She leaned over, her forearms resting on her thighs, her legs spread wide apart. The posture seemed a bit too informal since she was a very thin woman wearing an oversized housedress.

And she smoked. In fact, the entire house reeked from the odor of cigarettes, and the burn marks on her faded orange sofa and floral pillows confirmed that this was the case.

"I'm Melanie, and this is my son Jonathan. My mom said that you babysit."

"Yes, I do," she said, reaching out towards Jonathan and resting him at an odd angle against her left arm and thigh, as if she were cradling a football rather than an infant. Looking directly at me, she raised her right hand (it seemed as if she were holding an imaginary cigarette) and pointed to no one in particular. Then she got right to the point.

"I'll watch your baby for fifty dollars a week."

She didn't provide any qualifications for her position, nor was I in much of a position to ask her about her past experience with children. I was a teen, and I tried to be as deferential as possible considering her age. Her qualifications came down to just a few salient points: by the looks of the photos in her house, she was a grandmother; she was at home all day; she lived near a bus stop; and I could afford her. Fifty dollars a week was a lot for me, but it was less than what any formal, accredited daycare would have charged. I prayed right then and there that Jonathan's name would get to the top of the YMCA or campus childcare as soon as possible. Hopefully, Mrs. Cager would be a stopgap solution.

"Um, okay," I said.

From her hand gestures, I saw that she was still holding an imaginary cigarette, so I got up the nerve to ask the "burning question."

"Mrs. Cager, I'm sorry to ask, but do you smoke?"

"Just outside the house," she said, briefly flicking her wrist towards the window.

For a split second, I imagined her taking a long drag on a cigarette, blowing smoke towards Jonathan, and then flicking the butt out the window.

She asked me to follow her into the kitchen, where there was a pot of soup on a burner. She kept small playpens in both the living room and the kitchen, which, I suppose, was a good omen inasmuch as she had some concept of not leaving children unattended. The pot of grease on the stove reminded me of my grandmother's kitchen, but she was nothing like my grandma. Mrs. Cager wore gray, thinning hair in a tight bun on top of her head, and I wondered just how many years she had worn the same dress and hairstyle. She may have been a grandmother, but she wasn't one I could easily identify with.

* * *

Mom and I lived on the south side of Reno. The university was down-town, and Mrs. Cager's house was in the eastern section of the city. This meant I'd have to take multiple buses each day: a bus to Mrs. Cager's to drop Jonathan off, a bus to UNR, a bus to pick up Jonathan, and then a bus home. It would have been nice to have Mom give me a lift once in a while, but she wouldn't have done it since she was still the one-woman administrator of the LET MELANIE KNOW WHAT IT TAKES TO BE A MOTHER program. I knew the situation wasn't permanent, however, since my name would sooner or later rise to the top of the student housing list.

Things were tense at home since Mom constantly criticized me for the way I cared for Jonathan. I was either under-dressing him or over-dressing him; I was feeding him too much or too little; I was picking him up too much or too little when he cried. I was angry and resentful of my mother's approach since she had a car and her freedom, and as the saying went, talk was cheap. It's easy to criticize someone when you can walk away at any time. I had endured a great deal of stress and was coping far better than most in my situation, and I didn't need to be enrolled in Mom's teen mother educational program.

I talked to Ms. King, telling her of my frustration with all of the bus rides and my need to get into student housing. I felt as if I might be ready to graduate by the time my name surfaced on the housing list. As usual, she promised to make a few calls and see if there was a way to speed up the process. Meanwhile, I made $7.50 per hour in the work-study program. I filed papers, answered the phone, and signed students into the tutoring center. When there wasn't much to do, I used the time to study. Academi-cally, school was going okay since I'd been advised not to take too many credits, and my courses were similar to Advanced Placement classes, and as it turned out, my summer program at the Hughes Institute had more than prepared me for the basic courses I now took. I still had to stay focused and accept many new responsibilities, but I was easing into my coursework nicely.

A month later my name came up on the student housing list, although the news came with a downside. The housing wasn't conveniently located on campus, but rather north of Reno in a town called Stead, which was farther away from campus than my mother's apartment was. On the plus side, it represented inexpensive housing and freedom from Mom. If Darryl moved to Reno, we would have a place of our own. He would hopefully drive out in his car, with our own transportation making everything a lot easier each day. I immediately called him with the news about the housing opportunity.

"Melanie, let's get married," he said. "We can be a family, just like we talked about."

He'd caught me off guard. Marriage was a big step, but I would no longer be a single teen mother if I said "yes." I'd be a married woman with a husband and a son.

"I love you, Melanie," Darryl continued. "And I love Jonathan, too."

Those were words I needed to hear. I wasn't feeling loved given that I hadn't lost a significant amount of weight since the pregnancy. I was hovering around 200 pounds, and my abdomen was covered in stretch marks. Who would want me but Darryl? I needed help and support, and to hear of Darryl's affection for Jonathan was more than I had dared hope for.

I told my mother about my decision one day at the grocery store.

"How can you get married?" she asked. "You're only seventeen."

In a smart-alecky way, I informed her that I could get married according to state law if a parent or guardian granted consent.

"And just why would I grant you permission to do such a thing?"

"Because I'm going to be eighteen next month, and if you don't allow it, it's going to happen after my birthday in October. Darryl is coming, and we're going to live in student housing."

My mother reluctantly agreed, resigning herself to my stubbornness on the subject. Or she might have seen my impending marriage as a way to put an end to our current struggles each day. While I believed she enjoyed telling me what to do as part of her "training program," I believe she was at times weary of our butting heads and ironically yearned to have even greater freedom of movement.

Darryl arrived a week later on the bus. I wasn't sure why he hadn't driven his car out west, but at least he'd arrived sooner than I expected. I had the keys for our apartment, but I hadn't gone to see it yet. We'd be exploring it together.

Wasn't that what engaged couples did?

*　*　*

14

Mom secured a job for Darryl as a mechanic with the local dealership, which was welcome news inasmuch as I was desperate for even more financial and emotional support despite the generous grants obtained for me by Ms. King. We therefore moved into student housing fifteen miles north of Reno (and thankfully on the bus line). The housing units looked like old military barracks, and in point of fact, the area had been the site of a former Air Force base. The housing consisted of quadrangles of long cinderblock apartments laid out in a manner that a child might arrange rectangular cracker boxes when playing with Army action figures. Each apartment had two rooms connected by a small kitchen area. The accommodations were spartan, with no carpeting, molded cabinets, or accented bathroom fixtures, but it was someplace Darryl, Jonathan, and I could call home—and it didn't have my mother.

We decided to get married as soon as possible. Darryl had used the last of his money—his car, he said, had become too old to repair—so I took some work-study money to J.C. Penney's and purchased two simple gold wedding bands.

Next, we borrowed Mom's car—her resignation to the wedding extended to this rare loan—and decorated the back window with the traditional words "Just Married." Darryl, Jonathan, and I then headed into Reno for the ceremony. Mom was invited, but I knew better than to expect her attendance. Jonathan was in the back seat, peaceful and content, oblivious to what was going on. I wished that, in his serenity, he could give me some kind of sign, a validation, that I was doing the right thing. I knew that I didn't love Darryl, but I quickly pacified my conscience by reminding myself that this was more for Jonathan than anyone else. If I were more secure, then my son would be cared for better. As far as Darryl and I falling in love again, my seventeen-year-old mentality was tantamount to looking at our situation through rose-colored glasses. I thought it possible, and mere possibility was good enough for me to take the plunge if it meant a better life for Jonathan.

With Jonathan in my arms at the courthouse, I stood across from Darryl as we recited our vows. Everyone else there was a stranger, but I was now legally married. My heart was nevertheless torn. Was Jesus still looking down at us even now, knowing that I was making a marriage of convenience? Did he understand my desperate need for help? Had he witnessed all of my struggles? Would he strengthen us, helping us to make the marriage a true union of two souls? I thought the answer to all of these questions was "yes." God knew that, in my heart, I was hoping and praying for a miracle. He also knew that I was doing everything in my power to help make it happen and that I wanted the real thing. I think that's all any of us can ever do: try.

* * *

After spending $500 on the wedding rings, Darryl never wore his. He claimed it would get dirty because of the grease and grime from the mechanical work he did. While such a remark made it sound like he was working very hard every day, he complained ceaselessly that he was the only black man at the dealership, which he believed to be racist. He also said that his hands ached from working on hot cars all day and that he'd had enough of inhaling exhaust fumes. But hadn't he worked as a mechanic in Jackson? Didn't dirt, exhaust, and calloused hands come with the territory?

"I wish I could sit on my butt all day at some school like you do," he remarked one day.

Uneducated, Darryl had no idea of the rigors that college can present to a student. While my coursework wasn't burdensome yet, I still had to study in addition to taking care of Jonathan, working on campus, and riding what seemed an endless number of buses each day. How could he imagine that I had it easy? The world of books, ideas, and campus life was alien to Darryl.

Whenever I asked him for money, he grew annoyed. His facial muscles tensed as soon as I brought up the subject.

"I got to send home money to my mother. She ain't got me there, and money got to come from somewhere."

I'd asked Darryl to come to Reno because I thought I would get a little financial help among other things, but I was becoming suspicious as to where his paycheck was going. I doubted that any money was being sent to Jackson. He would go out at night, coming home late and smelling of alcohol. On the one hand, I relished these quiet moments when I didn't have to choose my words carefully for fear that he might lose his temper, plus I enjoyed the quiet, when I could sit at the table, rocking Jonathan to sleep while reading my chemistry textbook.

As time wore on, he came home later and drunker, and my suspicions were confirmed. Considering where we lived, I knew he was gambling our money away. "I'm going downtown for a bit," was a regular line he fed me in the early evenings as he groomed himself fastidiously in the manner of an ex-soldier, ironing his shirt and making sure that his appearance was perfect, from his hair to his shoes. If I questioned him about his nocturnal activities, he became angry and defensive.

"Look!" he would shout. "I've done come all this way for you. I had a good-paying job in Jackson. You ain't got nothin' to say to me. Besides, you don't know what I have to deal with at work."

I felt like I had two children instead of one.

* * *

We bought a car a few weeks later, an old Volvo that Darryl bought for $400 from the dealership where he worked. With money spent on both the car and gambling, our bank account was getting tight. While Darryl was a mechanic, we didn't even have enough money to purchase old parts from an auto junkyard so he could repair the Volvo, and Darryl would often use a coat hanger to keep parts from literally dropping onto the street as we drove. The car was falling apart, as was the marriage.

It was getting tough to scrape together a meal, so I swallowed my pride and went to the food pantry at school, where faculty, students, and staff would donate nonperishable items for other students. I chose a box of Hamburger Helper, a simple dish that would require only a little milk and ground beef in addition to the contents of the box.

I set the table, and dinner was ready when Darryl got home. He looked surprised.

"It's dinner!" I announced, beaming proudly.

He sat across from me, looking suspicious, as if I, a student with her head always buried in a book, might have stolen the meal. He took one bite before proclaiming, "This shit is nasty!"

I looked at the box sitting in the trash and saw that the expiration date was over a year old. I had gone to a lot of trouble to do something special, but nothing ever seemed to go right.

"You can't even cook!" he said, sneering. "I don't know why you tried. You don't do nuthin' around here. You're fat, and your ass looks like chewed up bubblegum. I'm going downtown to get me something to eat."

"Darryl, please don't go! I really tried so hard to—"

He turned around and snapped at me. "Tried hard to do what? You sit on your ass all day saying you're gonna to become a doctor. I got news for ya. You ain't gonna be shit."

Jonathan started to scream as Darryl's voice grew louder.

"Shut him up!" Darryl demanded. "Shut him up right now!"

I begged Jonathan to be quiet, but an infant cannot process the desperation of a mother being abused. To a baby, such a chaotic episode is nothing but blurry vision and meaningless sound. It's also the way such an episode appears to the abused mother. I felt as if I were in a horror movie, where reality becomes more and more distorted.

Darryl grabbed me by the neck and threw me roughly against the refrigerator, with cereal, bread, and other items tumbling to the floor, as if a small earthquake had hit the town of Stead. In a very real sense, it had.

Darryl's eyes were piercing as he gazed at me with a look of madness, freezing me as I stood straight as a pole against the refrigerator, his fingers wrapped around my throat. Was he going to choke me right in front of our son?

He left abruptly, not turning back. Gasping and relieved, I scooped up Jonathan and held him close. We both cried until we fell asleep.

* * *

Someone slapped my face early the next morning.

"Why ain't there no money in the account?"

The smell of alcohol mixed with the harsh, demanding words spoken above my face.

I was dazed after a deep, dreamless sleep in the wake of Darryl's attack the night before. Ironically, I was waking to another nightmare.

"You heard me," Darryl repeated. "Why ain't there no money?"

I wanted to say, "Because you gambled it all away," but I didn't want to precipitate another domestic earthquake. I was fairly sure my neighbors knew of our troubles, which was another source of embarrassment for me. A married female medical student knew of my situation because I'd confided in her, albeit in broad strokes, some of the details of my history with Darryl.

"I'm sorry, Darryl. I'm sorry there isn't any money. I'll get more—I promise. I'll go to financial aid and get a loan." I wasn't sure this was even possible, but I was desperate to avoid an encore of the previous evening's chaos.

The combination of sweat and alcohol emanating from Darryl's moist skin reminded me of the awful days in Jackson, sitting in his room beneath the picture of Jesus, his mother locked into her own peculiar world while watching mindless television. I tried to think of something else, tried to dissociate by thinking of chemistry or math equations—tried to think of anything but the drunken Darryl suddenly climbing on top of me for the purpose of sex.

He got up and left, leaving me to lie in bed, wondering what would happen next.

* * *

My eighteenth birthday had arrived on October 13, 1994. Darryl, following the pattern of most abusers, had treated me nicer in the past couple of weeks so as not to drive away the one person he knew would put up with his abusive behavior. The car was running—barely—and he was beginning to teach me how to drive around the lonely streets of Stead. I therefore went to school feeling pretty good on my birthday, hoping that he had planned something special for me later that day. I was now legally an adult.

Mom picked me up from Mrs. Cager's—she was more helpful now that I wasn't the perennial thorn in her side—and brought me home. I went in after she dropped me off and saw Darryl slumped in the sofa, watching TV with two forty-ounce beer cans next to him.

"What you doin' here?" he asked.

I was thinking the same thing about him. Why wasn't he at work?

"I decided to come home early since it's my birthday," I said. "I don't have to work on campus today."

"Oh, yeah, that's right," he said. "Happy birthday." He took a swig of beer and kept his attention focused on the television.

"Did you come home early for my birthday?" I asked him.

His answer was blunt. "No. As a matter of fact, I don't work there no more."

"What?"

"They fired me."

He said this with no more emotion than if he'd said, "It's warm outside."

It didn't take a rocket scientist to figure out what had happened. He wasn't just drunk—he was *a* drunk, an alcoholic—and he'd been unable to put in a sober day of work at the dealership.

"Oh," I said.

Tears gathered in the corners of my eyes. Why did they have to fire him on my birthday of all days? I realized in an instant, however, that he may have been fired days, or even weeks, earlier. He'd finally confessed simply because he'd gotten caught. I nevertheless hoped he had planned something on my birthday. He'd mellowed a bit, right?

"Darryl, Mom has Jonathan, and I was wondering what we're doing to celebrate my birthday."

"I don't know," he answered flatly. ""What you want to do?"

There was food in the house, but I didn't feel like making a meal and forcing conversation. I was eighteen, and the day called for something special.

"I'd like to get something at Service Merchandise," I said. "Can we go there?"

I had spotted a heart pendant at the store months before, and I really thought it would make a great birthday present.

"All right," he said.

We headed to the store, but Darryl handed me a hundred dollar bill and stayed in the car.

He wasn't showing a great deal of romance, but the hundred dollars would cover the price of the pendant, so I counted my blessings and went inside to the jewelry counter. The total price, with tax, was $107, so I used the few dollars I had in my purse to make up for the shortage. Putting the necklace on, I smiled as I saw my image in the glass counter. "Happy birthday, Melanie," I whispered to myself.

Outside, Darryl said nothing about my purchase.

"That didn't take long," he said. "Where's my change?"

I swallowed hard and paused. "There isn't any change. It was $99 plus tax."

I could have anticipated his reaction but for the fact that this was my birthday and he'd been a lot less angry with me lately.

"Didn't I just tell you I don't have a job? Who you trying to impress with that thing?"

His anger was starting to simmer. I'd grown used to the signs. I sat silently as he lectured me about how selfish I was and how he was fed up with "racist Reno and dead Stead."

When we got home, all I could think of was how glad I'd been that he hadn't ripped the pendant from my neck in the car. Now feeling ashamed of myself for spending so much money on myself, I crept into the bathroom, removed the pendant, and hid it. It had indeed cost too much, but I deserved it.

* * *

Darryl was still unemployed by November, and I doubted that he was seriously looking for another job at all.

When changing linen on a Saturday when Darryl wasn't home, I heard a clinking sound under the bed. Bending over, I saw about twenty empty beer cans wedged in the coils of the box spring. He'd promised to stop drinking on several occasions, but I knew that it wasn't going to happen, not even for Jonathan's sake. I was becoming bitter and resentful that he was taking the marriage so lightly. I'd given him every chance, but he didn't take his duties as father or husband seriously. For Darryl, having a family meant having a woman he could have sex with, get money from, and wail on when he was three sheets to the wind.

I was talking to Sarah on the phone when Darryl came home later that day.

"Get off the phone!" Darryl ordered.

I hoped Sarah hadn't heard the remark. I'd told her about Darryl's possessive and controlling behavior, although I didn't tell her about the physical abuse. I believe she suspected it, however.

I nodded to Darryl that I would wrap up the conversation.

"I said get off the phone *now*! When I say get off the phone . . ." To finish his sentence, he simply pulled the phone cord out of the wall.

Why was he so angry?

"You talk on the phone too damn much," he said. "I don't want to hear all that talk 'bout nothing."

"Darryl, I need friends. Sarah and I have classes together, and we need to talk about school."

"Friends? *I'm* your only friend. No one else cares about you. She just pretends to." He was yelling again, lecturing me as he marched up and down the hallway like a trapped lion.

I remained silent. I'd learned to keep my mouth shut to prevent his emotional earthquakes and their aftershocks. His ranting was interrupted by a knock on the door. It was the police.

"A concerned citizen called," said an officer. "Is everything okay here?"

I had a strong hunch that the "concerned citizen" was Sarah.

"Yes, officer" said Darryl. "Everything is just fine. No problem. Just a few words with the wife. That's all."

"Is there anyone else home?" the officer asked. "I'd like to speak to them as well."

"It's just my husband and my baby," I volunteered, my heart pounding until I could hear the blood in my ears.

They came in and asked Darryl a few more questions, and he talked his way out of the jam in the fashion of a true abuser. We'd had an argument. We were a young couple with a newborn. Small apartment and broken down car. Not a lot of money. Won't happen again. Yes, sir. No, sir. Thank you, sir.

The police hadn't been gone for more than five minutes before Darryl started yelling again. "You had your friend call the goddamned police! The damned police, Melanie?" He was angrier than ever. "She ain't no friend of yours, and you ain't never talkin' to her again."

"I won't ever talk to her again," I promised, willing to say or do anything to calm his wild temper.

I secretly prayed that the police would return to hear Round Two in progress, but there was no knock on the door.

Jonathan was screaming at the top of his lungs. Darryl picked him up in one swift motion that caused instant terror to flow through my veins.

"Darryl, please give him to me," I pleaded, opening my arms. "Please."

He threw Jonathan in my direction. My heart stopped as I caught my baby in mid-flight. I squeezed him tightly and kissed the top of his head. I hated Darryl and decided I would not allow him to hurt Jonathan again.

* * *

I was awakened at 2 a.m. Sleepily, I shuffled to the front door, wondering why Darryl didn't have his key. What I saw moderated the hateful feelings I'd harbored toward Darryl five hours earlier. He was covered in blood, as was my black and silver Raiders jacket. His white shirt was bright red, his face bruised and bloody. His lip was swollen, and one of his eyes was almost completely shut.

"What happened, Darryl?"

"Call 911."

I could barely understand him, and my fingers were shaking as I dialed the emergency number and told them of Darryl's condition, begging them to come immediately.

"I was jumped," Darryl said.

He paced back and forth, blood dripping to the floor, while I tried to listen to the operator, his body fueled by pure adrenaline. I got off the phone and put some ice on his swollen face as he told me what had happened.

"I took the bus downtown," he said. "When I came back, I got off the bus and five Mexicans walked up to me and asked for a cigarette. 'I ain't got no cigarette,' I told 'em, but then one of 'em got in my face. He got *too* close, so I punched him. That's when they all jumped me. I was outnumbered and thet started kickin' me."

That sounded like Darryl. Full of military bravado and drunken confidence, he thought he could take on anyone when in fact he was in over his head from the beginning of the encounter.

The ambulance showed up in a matter of minutes and took Darryl to the hospital, but not before my neighbors emerged, naturally curious as to what all the excitement was about. The sympathetic married medical student gave me a lift, the two of us following the ambulance in her car.

Darryl was diagnosed with bruised ribs, a broken nose, and missing teeth. I called Mom, who offered to come pick up Jonathan, who I had of course brought with me. I hoped Mom would stay since I felt so alone and couldn't ask my neighbor to keep vigil with me for the next several hours. I was eighteen, but I had no idea how to handle such a situation in the ER.

"What am I supposed to do, Mom?"

"Don't sign any papers," she shot back, "because all this is going to cost a lot of money. And he was brought to the hospital by an ambulance? They're not free, Melanie. They cost money, too. Don't sign anything."

Mom was giving me useless advice. I didn't know anything about the cost, but I knew that I had to sign papers for Darryl to be treated. Despite his inexcusable behavior towards me, I couldn't let him lie on a gurney, his face misshapen. He was Jonathan's father, if nothing else, and he needed care. What was my mother thinking? I suspect that Darryl's welfare was not high on her list of priorities.

As I ended my exchange with Mom on a payphone, I heard the tail end of conversation between Darryl and the police. An officer asked Darryl if he was in a gang.

"No, he's my husband," I said, interrupting. "The jacket is mine, and this is our son Jonathan. Darryl didn't do anything wrong. He was assaulted."

It was obvious that the officer assumed that, because of the jacket and our ethnicity, Darryl had street connections. Maybe he did, but I knew he wasn't in an actual gang. Even as I defended my husband to the police, I couldn't help but wonder if everything that had happened that night was karma, payback for the violent way Darryl had treated me in the kitchen. I wiped away the tears from my cheeks as I attempted to be a supportive wife.

Maybe this would bring us all closer.

* * *

15

It was my hope that Darryl would agree to counseling, and through the process of couples therapy learn that we could get through anything together. We could learn how much we needed each other, and perhaps he would even start going to church. He would learn that people had to rely on each other, and if he could assimilate this concept of community, he would come to understand that it was good for me to have friends. By the same token, he might learn that it wasn't good for him to always keep to himself except for when he hit the casinos.

I skipped classes the day after Darryl was assaulted so I could nurse him. I watched him sip clear liquids, such as milk, juice, and Gatorade, thinking to myself what a contrast he now presented to the strong, athletic young man I'd met in the parking lot of the Baptist church in Jackson, or even the aggressive man I'd had to contend with only a week earlier. He'd been laid low, and our roles had been reversed. He couldn't get through the day without me. Would such an experience be a sobering influence for him, both literally and figuratively.

I told Ms. King what had happened, omitting the causes behind Darryl's assault or information concerning his abusive behavior—I'd be too embarrassed (seemingly a constant emotion throughout the last two years of my life)—and she informed me about the Victims of Crime Fund, bankrolled by the state of Nevada. Knowing of my financially precarious situation, she said I shouldn't worry about hospital bills since Darryl would likely qualify for the program. The ER and ambulance expenses would be covered.

Unfortunately, the medical expenses didn't stop with Darryl's treatment at the ER. He would need oral surgery, plus an ENT doctor would be required to repair his broken nose. Since he wouldn't be able to work for weeks (possibly months), I once again experienced severe anxiety over financial concerns, but Ms. King reassured me that I could get loans for these aspects of his care as well. I didn't want to incur any debt since I was relying heavily on financial assistance of one kind or another, but I was in a bind. I felt increasingly guilty for asking Darryl to leave Jackson based on mere speculation that we might fall in love for the sake of Jonathan and my financial security. My starry-eyed optimism could have gotten Darryl killed.

I engaged in endless self-recriminations. If I had only been outside our apartment a few minutes before the assault, maybe the Mexican guys would have walked away. Maybe, maybe, maybe. If only had had done this or done that. I went over Darryl's condition a dozen times in my mind, and each time I felt responsible even though I knew from a rational standpoint that I had no control over his erratic activities or those of the group who had beaten him up. He shouldn't have been drinking and gambling, but as someone who was firmly co-dependant by this time, I erroneously assumed the responsibility and felt that I was not only to blame in some way, but that I could make everything better.

I still didn't love Darryl, but I felt sympathetic for what he was going through. I was indeed able to find an ear, nose, and throat surgeon, and he repaired Darryl's nose at reduced charges. The oral surgeon, however, told me that replacing Darryl's front teeth was cosmetic in nature and would not be covered by the Victims of Crime Fund. The cost, therefore, was prohibitive. Consequently, Darryl would run his tongue along his gums, complaining that he couldn't stand being snaggletoothed, as he termed it, but I could do nothing but tell him that we would save up in order to get the necessary oral surgery. To keep his beast in check, I even lied and told him how much I loved him.

Darryl's recuperation lasted a month, after which he claimed that he was always tired. Back on solid food, he ate and sat in front of the TV all day long, watching soap operas and game shows. With his alleged fatigue, he declined to look for work, playing the role of victim to the hilt even though he was fully capable of going out, buying a paper, and looking in the classifieds for a mechanic's position. The truth was that, now off his pain meds, Darryl had changed his liquid intake from Gatorade to beer.

Meanwhile, I continued to take Jonathan to Mrs. Cager's every morning. Leaving our son with Darryl wasn't an option since his volatility was always seething beneath the surface. I knew he was capable of changing from a quiet, sunny sky to a dark, menacing thunderstorm in a matter of seconds, and given his lethargy, he simply wasn't attentive enough to care for a young child. If Jonathan started to cry on any given day, I worried that Darryl might possibly injure his own son lest he be distracted from his soaps.

When I returned in the evening, Darryl was always sitting in the exact same spot as in the morning. As the Bible says, there was nothing new under the sun.

* * *

I went out to dinner at Applebee's with Sarah one evening. Darryl still harbored ill feelings toward Sarah, but he had resigned himself to allowing me a connection with her and other students owing to his own sense of guilt about the mugging, plus the fact that I'd taken care of him at a time when he himself couldn't. It was not a position he was used to being in. Begrudgingly, he granted me the extra space. Before leaving the apartment for dinner with Sarah, I left Darryl a note requesting that he clean up a bit since the apartment looked like the aftermath of a tornado. If Sarah gave me a ride home, I would be mortified if she saw the amount of trash scattered around the apartment thanks to Darryl's moratorium on life beyond our small apartment.

I told Sarah over dinner how embarrassed and frustrated I was about the way things were playing out with Darryl. She, after all, was the concerned citizen who had called the police when Darryl had gotten out of hand a month earlier, and she was someone I could talk to, relating even the sordid details of my marital relationship.

Sarah was firm and honest in her response, careful not to cross the boundaries that might endanger our friendship. "He's costing you a lot," she said, "and not just financially, but emotionally as well. Is it worth it? Why are you still with him when he treats you so badly?"

I understood the question all too well, but Sarah hadn't lived through the struggles I had, nor was she aware of the trade-offs I'd made to not only survive but also to get into college as a pre-med student. I knew she was very concerned about me, but she was part of the "regular" college scene, attending parties, dating, and living a more carefree existence. Except for shared experiences at school, we lived in two different worlds.

"He's my husband," I explained. "This wouldn't have happened if I hadn't asked him to come to Nevada and move in with me."

My answer had little effect on Sarah's assessment of the situation. She tried to persuade me to leave Darryl, but my guilt was too heavy to consider such a radical step.

She gave me a ride home, and the apartment was as messy as when I'd left. Darryl was slumped on the couch as usual, absorbed in some television show. Sarah hugged me, kissed Jonathan on the cheek, and whispered in my ear, "Be safe." She and I could both feel the tension from being in the same room with my husband. His irritation at her presence in the apartment was palpable.

I was no longer buying into Darryl's constant spiel about being too tired from injuries. If he wasn't out looking for a job, the least he could have done was pick up the trash he'd strewn throughout the rooms, taking all of thirty minutes to tidy up so that I could bring a friend inside without being ashamed of my home. It was that night that something in me said, "Enough." I looked at the beer cans, the pizza boxes, and the dishes piled high in the sink and told Darryl, "I'm going to sleep in the other room." I had no desire to be with him. In retrospect, Sarah's words had made more of an impact than I thought.

"No you ain't!" Darryl countered. He followed me into the other room, slipped on the floor, and upon standing up, pulled me around sharply and hit me on the cheek.

"You act like the only one who's tired around here. Don't you *never* ask me to clean up for your friends! You need to do what a spouse is 'spose to do."

The beast within had been unleashed.

He demanded I return to the other room, telling me how much he'd sacrificed to be near me. He then launched into a maniacal lecture that I knew could be the harbinger of more domestic violence. He was drunk and out of control.

"You clean this shit up!" he demanded. "That's what a wife does!"

Hoping to avoid another visit from the police, I began picking up food wrappers and cans and placing them in the trash. As I did, I thought how terrible it would be to come home to an empty apartment each day. I didn't know how to fix a running toilet or a leaky faucet, but another part me wanted Darryl gone for good, and that part of myself was gaining power.

As I continued my chores, I wondered if Jonathan would turn out to be like his father. Would he learn through observation that this was how a father acted? Would he treat women as Darryl did? I was growing angrier with each passing second. My finals were coming up, and becoming a doctor suddenly seemed an unrealistic goal if I continued on the same path. I couldn't sustain this type of lifestyle for another seven years. Indeed, at eighteen, I felt old and worn out.

Deep in my gut, I couldn't rationalize Darryl's irresponsible behavior any longer or lie to myself about the consequences of living with him.

* * *

A letter arrived not long after that horrible night of listening to my lazy husband school me in the duties of a wife, a letter that would change my life. It was from the Reno Housing Authority. My name had been on their waiting list since I'd moved to Reno in May. Now, several months later, they had a unit available for me in an area called Raleigh Heights, which was closer to town than Stead. If Darryl started working again, however, I wouldn't qualify for the public housing, plus I'd originally signed up for an apartment for two, not three.

In February of 1995, therefore, I had to make a decision of the utmost importance. Raleigh Heights was more upscale, with landscaping and playgrounds. The units themselves were more like town homes, and the move would be good for both me and Jonathan. Darryl, on the other hand, had resumed his nightly trips downtown to the casinos and was drinking heavily again. The housing authority was only going to hold my place for a week, so I needed to give them an answer as quickly as possible. The decision, as it turned out, was made for me.

Darryl returned home at eleven-thirty one evening and demanded sex even though I was studying for a psychology test the following day. I realized that my choice was between my studies and a life with Darryl, the quality of which wasn't going to change—not ever. I let him climb on top of me, but this time I didn't focus on math equations to dissociate myself from his unwanted sexual advance. Rather, I thought of how and when I was going to leave him. I was resigned to the fact that my bold experiment to create a family had failed. It was time for me to protect myself, my dreams, and most of all, Jonathan.

I called Mom the very next day and told her that I'd like to stay with her for a while and would be coming over after school. I hadn't shared any of the details of Darryl's domestic abuse—I didn't want to listen to a bunch of "I told you so's—but my mother almost certainly had more than an inkling as to what was going on. Her only response was, "That's a smart decision, Melanie." I appreciated the brevity of her answer.

Darryl called my mother's home that evening, begging me to come home.

"I can't," I replied. "I have to study."

"You can study at home," he said, crying. "You need to come back home *now*."

I hung up and tried to resume studying. He had apologized before, moderating his behavior briefly in order to keep me under control. This time, I wasn't going to place any faith in his ability to change.

He knocked on my mother's front door half an hour later. My mother opened the door, blocking the entrance.

"I need to speak to my wife," he said.

"She's not available right now," Mom answered tersely.

Darryl knew better than to tangle with my mother. Even in Jackson, he'd been aware that she was a force to be reckoned with. She would have shut the door in his face without hesitation. If he would have created a scene, she would have called the police in a New York minute.

The following day, Mom paid two of her male friends $160 to rent a Uhaul truck and pick up my things in Stead. She wanted to provide a little muscle to help me move—plus protection as well.

When we arrived in Stead, Darryl folded his arms around me and cried. "Melanie, you don't have to do this. We can get counseling."

He was a day late and a dollar short in his suggestion that we seek professional help.

"No," I said, holding back my tears so he wouldn't think I was afraid of him. I also didn't want to let him know that I was emotionally vulnerable even though I'd made a definitive decision. I needed to show strength and demonstrate that I was no longer going to be manipulated by empty promises. I had to look forward.

"My mom told me to give this to you," I said, handing him an envelope.

"What's this?" he asked, perplexed.

"Mom sold the Volvo and used the money to buy you a one-way train ticket back to Jackson. *That's* what's in the envelope."

Darryl stood there, glaring at me in disbelief as the movers diligently removed my belongings from the apartment. I doubted that he believed I possessed the resolve to stand up to him.

"You remember one thing," Darryl said, knowing that he'd been bested. "You tell Jonathan who it was that sent me away. You tell him I wanted to be a father to him, but you wouldn't allow me to."

I made no reply. I walked toward the parking lot, where the moving van was getting ready to leave. My life in Stead was over.

* * *

16

Darryl did not go quietly into that good night. He was persistent, if nothing else. He called my mother's house every day, begging to speak to me, begging for a chance to lure me back to our old apartment. I myself was reluctant to answer the phone, and I was glad to have Mom handle the situation in true Dorothy Watkins fashion. I was afraid of being sucked back into Darryl's twisted world of unpredictable behavior, especially when his words echoed in my mind: *You tell Jonathan who it was that who sent me away*. Regardless of what Darryl had done, it was hard knowing that he would never again live with his father. But with school and Jonathan to tend to, I didn't need the added distraction of Darryl to cloud my thoughts and resurrect my self-recriminations. I wanted a divorce so as to gain a sense of closure. Fortunately, his calls became less frequent, and then stopped altogether. Darryl knew he wasn't going to get past the gate-keeper: my mother.

I looked through the yellow pages and saw ads for a dizzying array of divorce lawyers. I called twenty at random, relating my story to each one: I'd made a dreadful mistake and urgently needed to move forward in life. It was interesting to hear myself from an objective viewpoint telling my story in a dispassionate, business-like manner, with no pleading or emotion. (Was I channeling my mother?) Something must have come across in my voice since I found a sympathetic ear on the other end of the line on call number twenty-one. The lawyer said he'd take my case on a pro-bono basis without charging me the customary fees for a divorce proceeding. I would only be responsible for fees for notary services and copying documents. I was appreciative for the attorney's willingness to handle my case since I not only wanted to be legally free of Darryl, but wanted my maiden name back as well. It came as a pleasant surprise that I didn't have to contact Darryl at all. All that was required under Nevada law was to run three consecutive ads in the newspaper.

The swiftness with which events happened in my life was almost too much to mentally assimilate. I was pregnant at sixteen, married at seventeen, and divorced at eighteen. At least the divorce, unlike situations involving school, public assistance, or medical care, was not a gauntlet I had to run. It was simple and painless.

For me, that represented a paradigm shift in my life. Would the luck hold out?

* * *

Mom's hired muscle that had helped me leave Stead also helped me move into the public housing at Raleigh Heights. The unit was nothing that was going to make *Better Homes and Gardens*—there was no carpeting, the walls were a generic beige, and there were no ornamental touches in the two-story townhouse—but it definitely represented a step up from the barracks atmosphere in Stead. Outwardly, the area looked like any other town home community one might see across the United States. It was also on the bus line and ten miles closer to downtown Reno, so all in all, my situation had improved drastically. Darryl was no longer a threat to my safety (or my son's), and Jonathan now had a room with enough storage to accommodate all the things that kids need.

Even though living in Raleigh Heights represented a stigma inasmuch as it was public housing, I felt that my spirit was breathing a deep draft of refreshing spring air in May of 1995. I was wrapping up my second semester at UNR, which had been harder than the first and had gone beyond anything I'd picked up in AP courses in high school, and I also enjoyed talking with neighborhood kids at the playground on the Heights as Jonathan got to play with other children, something that had been lacking in his life.

Additionally, Jonathan was approved for a childcare scholarship at the YMCA, which meant that Mrs. Cager's services would no longer be required. Although her care of Jonathan had never presented a problem, nor had there ever been even a minor incident while Mrs. Cager had been his caregiver, I had always worried that she was smoking in the house, exposing Jonathan to second-hand smoke or a possible firehazard.

The wind was most certainly at my back. I received a $2,500 scholarship for my sophomore year from the Nevada Women's Fund, a scholarship organization specifically for female Nevada residents. It was snowing less, and the weather in general was more moderate. Things were turning around in so many areas of my life. Still something was missing: someone to share the good times with.

* * *

Despite my good fortune in 1995, I nevertheless experienced a certain amount of conflict as a young mother trying to make it through college with grades good enough for admittance to graduate school. Would this struggle continue until I could graduate with an M.D. behind my name? There had to be something more. I wanted to have a kind, reliable husband, someone who would also be a good father to Jonathan. I sometimes thought with envy of the medical student's wife who had driven me to the hospital the night Darryl had been attacked in Stead. She and her husband were a loving couple, and her husband's attentiveness served to reinforce the reality that all men weren't like Darryl. But who would be interested in *me*?

I weighed 220 pounds and felt like used goods. When studying, I constantly snacked on junk food rather than anything healthy. It was cheaper and slightly addictive. Between Jonathan and my studies, I didn't have time to cook or even heat up TV dinners, which were unappetizing anyway. The "freshman fifteen" had turned into the "freshman fifty." Who would want to date a single woman with a child, a woman who lived to study and (given my financial assistance and scholarships) studied to live in a very real sense?

* * *

Some of my neighbors would babysit for me sometimes, and at other times, I reciprocated the favor, happy that Jonathan would have further interactions with other kids.

I was a homebody, afraid to even attempt having a social life, but three of my friends convinced me to go out with them to a hip-hop club on one of evenings when I'd lined up a sitter for Jonathan. I accepted their invitation with a great deal of trepidation since I felt frumpy, like a divorced nerd.

When we arrived at the club, I was totally intimidated and stood against the wall, feeling as if everyone could see right through me and recognize me for the socially inept person that I was. I still couldn't drive—the beat-up Volvo was now history—so I was resigned to the fact that I would have to endure the status of wallflower until our driver was ready to leave, whenever that might be. My friends could club until the early hours of the morning. My thoughts, on the other hand, were mainly focused on whether Jonathan was okay and if I would be able to get back home at a decent hour and relieve the babysitter. I stood by myself, sipping on a cola, wondering when I would be able to climb into bed and put the night behind me.

"Is there some place you have to be?" asked a male voice.

I looked up to see a man standing before me. He was tall and handsome in a boyish way, with dimples that were evident even in the darkness of the nightclub.

"Uh, no," I answered. "I'm just waiting for my friends."

I was nervous, but in a hopeful way. My heart was racing. Was this man making idle conversation or was he actually interested in me? Was he making a polite, gentlemanly overture to me, Melanie Watkins, oversized pre-medical student?

"Why aren't you dancing?" he asked.

I had only been to high school dances, as well as a few clubs when I used to sneak out at night with Darryl back in Jackson. Mingling in a crowd wasn't my forte.

"I don't know," I replied. I looked away, unsure of what to say. I was caught off guard. There were dozens of other girls in the club, long-haired girls who were pretty and thin. Following the advice of my friends, I was wearing a black blouse, which had a slimming effect, and I'd accessorized it with my heart pendant and some gold hoop earrings. I even had on my favorite lip gloss, but all of these minor attempts to draw attention from my weight didn't change the fact that I was "plus-sized." Why was this man talking with me when so many slender, beautiful young women were available?

"Come on," said the young man, pulling my hand gently as he led me to the dance floor. I couldn't remember how long it had been since I'd danced with anyone, but I was a bit dizzy from the attention I was getting. Was this a dream?

I learned snippets of information about my dance partner as we shouted in each others' ears when the music occasionally dropped a few decibels. His name was Albert, and he lived in Herlong, California, an hour north of Reno. Originally from South Carolina, he was in the military police and wanted to become a regular police officer.

Military? An alarm bell sounded in my mind. Darryl had been in the Army Reserve when I'd met him in Jackson, and I wondered for a split second if all my good luck would always be overshadowed by destiny repeating itself. Why couldn't Albert have been a law student?

But I was getting way ahead of myself, panicking for no reason. Still, I remained somewhat guarded. I told him I was about to start my sophomore year at the university, although I omitted the fact that I had a child, lived in public housing, and was a pre-med student. I doubt that he wanted to date a bookworm. Most of all, I omitted that I'd been married. For those brief moments on the dance floor, I wanted to pretend that I was like my friends, without a care in the world, someone who went from party to party. And why shouldn't I? I would never see this guy again, right?

I was amazed, however, when Albert asked for my phone number at the end of the evening. He wanted to see me again. I didn't quite know what to expect, but I was walking on air, and I gave him my contact information.

My girlfriends drove me home. I think I had a slight smile on my face for the rest of the evening.

* * *

17

I was excited when Albert called me a few days later to talk about music, movies, and his travels with the Army. Most of all, he spoke of how close he was to his family in South Carolina. I still declined to tell him about Jonathan—the time and place for such a disclosure would present itself. I wanted him to get to know me so that he didn't feel he was taking on too much by investing time in our relationship. At the end of the conversation, he asked me to go see the movie *Dangerous Minds*.

My thoughts were racing since I hadn't had more than a handful of isolated dates, none of which evolved into any kind of relationship. At school the next day, my girlfriends wanted to know all the details, with Erica and Danielle, two roommates on campus, volunteering to babysit Jonathan. I didn't think they had much experience in caring for infants, but Mom wasn't going to baby sit so that I could have a social life—that hadn't changed—and I didn't want to ask my neighbor two weeks in a row, so we made plans for Erica and Danielle to pick up Jonathan at seven in the evening on Friday, with Albert due to arrive at seven-thirty. I'd greet him at the door but wouldn't let him in lest he see stacks of Pampers and Jonathan's toys. If the evening went well, maybe I would find the right moment to tell him I was a parent.

When Friday evening came, I took special care to blow dry and straighten my naturally curly hair. I was feeling pretty, as well as light and energetic. Then I looked at the clock and panicked. It was 7:15 and Erica and Danielle hadn't arrived. I called them, but there was no answer, which was just as good. If they had answered, there was no way they would be able to make it on time.

There was a knock on the door at 7:25. Was it Erica or Albert? There was nothing to do but open the door and see how things played out.

Albert stood before me, roses in hand, a sweet, slender man with dark chocolate skin. I was flustered, but not to the extent that I forgot how excited I was that such a man was interested in me.

"Um, hi, Albert. I . . ."

The headlights of Erica's car appeared. I didn't know whether to be relieved that my friends were finally here or angry that they were so late. I grabbed Jonathan, baby bag, car seat, and, walking past Albert, brought them to my friend's car. I was so nervous that I thought my sweat would cause my hair to curl up again.

"Hey, Mel," they said nonchalantly.

I didn't have time to tell them chapter and verse on how to care for Jonathan, which was frustrating since all parents leave a few instructions specific to their child before handing over care to a babysitter. It was too late to call the date off, so I gave them Mom's telephone number and walked back toward Albert, who had taken everything in stride. He was grinning.

"What was that all about?" he asked calmly.

I briefly considered lying to him in order to enjoy a carefree night, but that wouldn't have been fair to Albert.

"My friends had to pick up my son Jonathan so we could go out tonight," I answered.

"You have a son?" He smiled in disbelief. "Why didn't you tell me?"

It must have seemed odd that I had omitted such an important detail from our initial conversations despite Albert's constant talk about the importance of his family in South Carolina.

"Where is his father?" Albert didn't ask the question in an accusatory manner. He remained very unflappable, as if the situation wasn't all that unusual. I nevertheless didn't feel like spoiling the evening with information about my past.

"Albert, let's get going. We don't want to be late for the movie."

I smiled and sighed simultaneously while placing the flowers in a vase in the kitchen, wondering how much I should tell him—and when.

Albert continued to act like a perfect gentlemen, opening the car door so I could slide into the passenger seat. His behavior was in stark contrast to Darryl's, who had pulled up to Service Merchandise on my birthday, left the motor running, and declined to get out while I bought my heart pendant.

"Jonathan's father isn't around," I said, looking at my red nails that I'd polished earlier. "We aren't together anymore. He lives in Mississippi."

"So it's just you and Jonathan?"

"Yes. My mother lives in South Reno and helps out sometimes, but mostly it's just us." I paused, thinking of how to change the subject. "So have any of your friends seen this movie yet?"

"Yeah," Albert replied. "One of the guys said it was pretty good."

Halfway through the movie, Albert reached over and placed his hand over mine. The moment was all that mattered. If Albert's thoughtfulness and affection lasted only one evening, I would be fine with that. I even allowed myself to stop worrying if Jonathan was doing okay with Erica and Danielle.

We grabbed some fast food after the movie. Watching him eat his chips, I noticed that he wasn't arrogant or overconfident. He was simply comfortable being himself.

Albert surprised me by offering to pick up Jonathan and take us home, which raised my opinion of him even further. Not only had he taken my news in stride, but he was already offering to help out with babysitting logistics.

"Thanks for the lift." I said. "I don't even know how to drive."

"I'll teach you," he said.

With just three short words, he was telling me that he wanted to continue seeing me and that he was okay with my being a mother. I looked out of the window, feeling my eyes tear up.

* * *

Organic chemistry, known as O-Chem, is the weed-out class all pre-med students must take. If they can't make it through O-Chem-, they most likely don't have what it takes to handle the entire pre-med curriculum. In addition to the course textbook, students use molecular models in order to examine structures three dimensionally to see how carbon, hydrogen, and helium bond in different ways. Despite giving the class my all and attending many tutoring sessions given by teaching assistants for the Harvard-educated Dr. Tam Chang, my first exam grade was a 55 out of 100. I'd failed.

I felt as if I had let both myself and Albert down. After two months of dating, Albert and I were officially a couple, and he was my rock. He came over on the weekends, watching Jonathan or taking him to the park while I constantly studied. He enjoyed our part-time family life and even followed up on his promise and taught me to drive. Despite his help, I'd bombed the exam big-time.

During one of his weekend visits, I told him that I'd failed my grade on the test.

"You've been studying quite a lot," he remarked.

"I know, and I don't know how I can possibly study any harder."

This was more than a rhetorical statement since my migraines had returned due to the constant stress of school. The frequency of their onset was less, but they interfered with my day-to-day activities.

As we were eating Chinese food, he lifted his fork, took a bite of shrimp-fried rice, and said, "Well, why don't you just quit?"

Albert's remark was not tendered in an insulting way or in the fashion of one of Darryl's ultimatums, but it was obvious that my boyfriend just didn't "get it."

I put down my chopsticks. "Quit?" I didn't doubt his good intentions in making the recommendation, but was he a quitter? I thought military personnel were made of sterner stuff.

"Yes," he reiterated. "If the program is stressing you out so much, why not do something else?"

Albert didn't have a degree. He was a blue-collar man who knew that school wasn't for him. He was practical and matter-of-fact. It was a question of my Type-A personality bumping against his Type-B. It was sophistication versus a down-home mentality, chopsticks versus a fork. It was nevertheless disconcerting that he'd made the suggestion.

"This is something all pre-med students go through," I explained. "The other students are just as stressed as I am. If you want to be a doctor, you don't quit just because you have a tough class."

I was worried that he might try to give me a Dorothy Watkins-type speech, recommending that I become a nurse instead.

"Sometimes I think you care more about school than me," he said in his non-threatening voice.

He meant well, but now I was seeing the first red flag in our relationship. A bit of jealousy was coming out on his part. How could I convince him that we'd have a better life in the future, or that once we were married, we'd look back and realize that all the hard work was worth it? I needed him to cover my back one hundred percent and to believe in my goals.

"Am I the girl you want to be with, Albert?" I asked.

"For the rest of my life," he answered without missing a beat.

To be supportive, I took Jonathan to Albert's base in Herlong one weekend so we could watch him play football. The entire time, I worried about how much time I was losing to my studies, especially O-Chem. Maybe it was true. Maybe I did care more about studying and my ultimate goals than about being with Albert.

* * *

Over a period of many months, Tonya and I had begun to reconcile our differences through brief phone calls as time and money would allow. Having raised Jonathan for almost two years, I was in a better position to understand the difficulties Tonya had faced in being a single mother and raising Sloane. We became friends again during these conversations, although Tonya didn't let me forget that she was "the big sister." Her advice regarding Albert, for example, was "Stay focused." It was her way of telling me not to get pregnant. I assured her that I had obtained Depo Provera at the local student clinic and that I wasn't going to let anything deter me again from my academic pursuits. Still, Tonya believed that Albert was my rebound relationship given that my relationship with Darryl had been such a disaster. Her belief was that I shouldn't fall for the first guy who treated me with kindness. Perhaps my sister had more objectivity than I did, but I felt that, all things considered, Albert was a positive influence for Jonathan and me.

Mom was not fully behind the relationship either, even though she didn't have to watch Jonathan as much now that Albert was taking up the slack in the babysitting department.

"You let him spend all his time over there," she said. "He gets free food, free lodging, free TV, and free sex. You know how those military men are! They have girls everywhere—at home, at the base, at a city near where they are stationed."

Had Mom said "sex"? Well, it didn't take a rocket scientist to figure out that Albert and I had sex since he stayed over on weekends, and Mom never held anything back. But I didn't think Albert was being unfaithful. Why didn't she want to see me happy? How long would she lecture me with her Dorothy Watkins "life lessons"?

"He has his own place at the base, Mom," I said, "but it's an hour's drive to Herlong, so it's easier for him to stay over on the weekends."

I naturally didn't succeed in changing my mother's thinking.

* * *

"What will medical school be like?" Albert asked me one night, his head resting in my lap.

I couldn't sugarcoat the answer. Besides studying, I was still working many different jobs, and school was about the only subject pre-med students discussed. The curriculum was intense.

"It's going to to be very difficult, Albert. Harder than my work as an undergrad."

"I miss my family," he said, abruptly changing the subject.

Albert had grown up on a farm in a very close knit family in Gadsden, South Carolina. He often spoke of his family eating dinner together, while pigs and chickens wandered in the backyard of his home. His father and mother, four brothers, and an aunt and uncle all lived together in several trailers on their property. It made me think back to my grandparents near Shreveport. Could Albert and I be like them, married for decades in modest dwellings with farm animals scurrying about? It was a lifestyle far removed from the one I was living in Reno and on campus. I couldn't imagine my career leading me to Albert's very own version of Mayberry, but his hitch with the military would be up in April of 1996, and a decision would have to be made fairly soon.

"I can't stay here," he confessed. "I feel like my life is on hold."

On hold? Weren't we growing as a couple?

"Don't they have a medical school in South Carolina?" he continued.

There it was, out in the open. He wanted me to live on the farm with his family.

"Are you serious?" I asked.

"I want you to come to South Carolina when you're finished this May. My family will help you out."

As always, the idea of being part of a family was a powerful inducement to me, but hadn't I had enough of the south? Hadn't I moved enough already? And I'd had far too many people in my life promising to "help me out." I didn't even know his parents, and the idea just didn't resonate with me. Besides, many of my academic credits might not transfer after all of the hard work I'd put into them. I told him I'd think about it, although it seemed too much to consider since the Christmas holidays were fast approaching.

I hadn't seen Tonya since before Jonathan was born. I told Albert that I missed my family, too, and that as much as I'd love him to accompany Jonathan and me to Phoenix, we couldn't afford an extra airline ticket.

"No sweat," he said. "I'll drive us."

His sweet disposition seemed to have no end. He was willing to drive sixteen hours from snowy Reno to Phoenix with a child in the back seat. Was it too much for me to sacrifice a bit and at least consider moving to his home. After all, he wasn't telling me that I couldn't be a doctor, just that he valued his family. What more could anyone want than a mate who valued family so much?

* * *

I pulled a B in O-Chem and vowed to do everything in my power to get an A in the spring semester. But Jonathan seemed inconsolable, crying almost all day, or so it seemed. Was I a bad parent? I felt incompetent and lonely, and his crying and my studying were naturally incompatible.

Against the backdrop of my self-doubt, the Nevada Women's Fund asked me to speak at one of their events, believing that potential donors would be impressed by hearing how their money was put to such good use. I was one of their major success stories given the struggles I'd overcome.

When the time came, I took a deep breath and shared my story. As usual, I omitted details about Darryl, but I did tell them that I was a teenage mother and that I appreciated every bit of their $2,500 scholarship. I received a standing ovation, which made me feel awkward since I didn't think I'd accomplished very much considering all that was still on my plate.

After my talk, a thin, confident woman in a tailored pantsuit approached me.

"Melanie, my name is Alice Arndt, and I have a son who is a little older than yours. Your story was very touching, and I'd like to help you."

I didn't know what to say other than, "Um, thanks. That's really cool."

She gave me directions to her house—I knew how to drive but didn't have a car—and when she saw the puzzled look on my face, she asked where I lived and made arrangements to stop by.

She showed up a few days later in a big truck loaded with several bags of clothes and toys. The clothes were stylish and had been barely worn. Indeed, some still had the original store tags attached. Many of the outfits were from a store called Gymboree, a store I'd seen at the mall but never stepped foot in because it was too pricey.

"When is Jonathan's birthday?" my benefactor asked.

"May 7th."

"What do you think he'd like for his birthday?"

It was hard to formulate an answer when she'd already given me so much.

"You don't have to, Ms. Arndt! Really, this is enough."

"Alice!" she said, smiling. "Call me Alice!"

"Ms. Alice, this is more than enough," I stated gratefully.

"Just Alice!"

She took a piece of paper from her purse and wrote the words JONATHAN'S WISH LIST at the top. She then handed me the paper, along with her pen.

Wow and praise God, I thought.

I jotted down the word "tricycle" since I thought all pre-schoolers should have one.

"Are you sure that's all?" she asked, taking back the paper.

"That's it," I said.

But Ms. Arndt wasn't quite finished. She continued as if she hadn't heard me. "Let's see," she said, wetting the tip of the pen with her lips. "He'll need a helmet, knee pads, a bell, and everything that a young boy on a bike needs for protection and fun."

I looked at Jonathan and smiled, then glanced at Ms. Arndt. She was a generous career mom and seemed to have it all. I hoped that I, too, could be as professional and generous in the years ahead.

* * *

I sometimes felt as if I was standing still while the world was spinning around me. I was spending so much time studying O-Chem that my test scores for microbiology and history were in the C range, and C students didn't get into medical school. I went into the bathroom one day and cried until I thought I would vomit. Despite the intense pressure on all pre-med students, it seemed as if all of my peers were having fun but me. My nose was in a book constantly, but what did I have to show for it but mediocre grades? I was also very tired on most days. I went to sleep early, hitting the bed as soon as Jonathan was down for the night, but the alarm sounded at

4:00 a.m. so that I could study at the living room table in the early morning quiet. I could have used the extra sleep, but if I didn't get into med school, what would I do with my degree?

I was frequently irritated and angry—angry at Albert for being so relaxed, angry at my friends for having enjoyable lives, angry at Jonathan for taking up so much of my time, and angry at my mother for continually reminding of all that I was supposedly doing wrong. It was a classic case of stress producing displaced anger, but I was only human. Given my work and study load, I was no longer finding any joy in Jonathan, Albert, or school. What I was living through was a far cry from the heady days of my days in the Hughes program. I even had to work during spring break, when the campus was nearly deserted, enhancing my feeling of isolation. I often thought that if I owned a car, I would simply take I-80 east and drive, not caring where I might end up. I felt stupid for thinking that I could handle everything.

Things didn't get any better when Albert announced that his younger brother had become a father. Albert felt that he was being left behind in his quest for the kind of family life his parents had. He had a timeline for starting his own brood, and I wasn't at all sure I could follow it. He even felt that Jonathan's shyness—he wasn't talking very much yet—was attributable to his not having a baby brother or sister. Why couldn't he let the subject of family go for a while so I could keep up with my coursework?

It was on "dead day," when all students prepare for final exams, that I brought some cupcakes to Jonathan's daycare at the YMCA. The director of his program approached and asked me if we could have a few words together.

"We're concerned about Jonathan," she said. "He doesn't appear to be speaking as many words as he should."

My first thought was that Albert had been correct. Being an only child, Jonathan needed more interaction with other children. He was indeed a loner, and he often conducted conversations with himself, although he didn't use real words as much as sounds in the form of songs. I had no idea how many words a child was supposed to know by age two. As the old adage goes, babies don't come with an instruction manual.

"We'd like to administer some tests at a special children's clinic," the director said. "He may be socially or developmentally delayed."

I was very worried but retained my composure. In fact, I was almost defensive given that I'd moved heaven and earth to keep Jonathan and care for him, and the idea that something might be wrong with him would only make me feel less adequate as a parent.

The woman handed me some consent forms to sign, which I did.

* * *

I called Mom to inquire about my speech when I was growing up and if she'd noticed anything unusual about Jonathan.

"Melanie," she said, "if you would just spend more time with him and read to him more, he wouldn't have any speech problems at all. That's all it is."

Mom had hit a raw nerve. It was allegedly my fault since I wasn't spending enough time with him. I decided that her advice was worth exactly what I'd paid for it: nothing.

Having been stressed out by my mother, I continued to work my many jobs and satisfy various prerequisites for getting into medical school, such as community service and participation in leadership activities at school. A great GPA wasn't good enough. For example, I'd received a $500 community service scholarship from UNR, but the money came with a heavy price. I just couldn't fit everything into a single day.

* * *

Albert was very supportive when Jonathan's evaluation revealed that he suffered from a speech delay. He required sessions with a speech therapist, and Albert was generous with his time to make sure Jonathan got to his appointments.

It was at this time, as he provided me much-needed help, that he gave me a brochure about the University of South Carolina. The out-of-state tuition was incredibly expensive, and it seemed the height of folly to give up all of my scholarships at the University of Nevada in order to move to South Carolina, where everything would be an unknown variable. Was Albert's "farm family" going to foot the bills for my medical training? Did they even have the means to do so, assuming they had the inclination?

I discussed the matter with Ms. King, who gently reminded me that she had worked hard to get me started at UNR and keep me there. I felt a bit ashamed, and I couldn't deny that she'd been instrumental in helping me get established at the university, but there were so many other factors to consider. What if I never got married or had more children? The statistics were grim when it came to single African American women raising children without a father. Because of socio-economic and educational factors, it wasn't easy to find an African American man who was as interested in family as Albert was. What good was it to become a doctor if I had no one to share my success with?

My migraines continued to parallel my stress level, and so I signed up for counseling at school, where I was assigned a psychology graduate student (who practiced under supervision). I needed to talk with someone neutral, although I had no idea how the counseling process worked. The grad student was a young overweight woman who was quite average looking, whereas I believed that all therapists must surely lead perfect lives and know exactly what to do and say in all situations. If my grad student knew all the answers, why was she overweight?

I related my experiences as a teen mom and the hardships I was currently facing. Her very simplistic answer was that I was depressed, a conclusion I could have come up with on my own. The remedy? She told me to eat better, exercise, work on stress management and relaxation techniques, and not to work or take classes during the summer. This was great advice in an ideal world, but when was I supposed to find the time to exercise? And how could I get by without working? She didn't *get* my life because she didn't *have* my life. Her expectations were unrealistic.

I figured that God had to be a better counselor than the hapless grad student, so I started attending a local church. Sundays were precious study days, but I reasoned that if I gave more time to God, he would give me more guidance. And it felt good to pray, asking God to carry some of my burdens. I imagined my grandparents saying, "Hold to God's unchanging hand."

* * *

The Reno Housing Authority became suspicious that Albert was living with me because his car was always in front of my town house. They monitored such situations carefully since many individuals tried to move in with friends living in public assistance units, and the housing authority wasn't inclined to support more people than it had approved. Our living situation, therefore, had to be resolved. Since Albert's time in the military was virtually up, Sarah suggested I fly out to South Carolina and get a feel for Albert's family and the surrounding area before I commit to anything. I didn't want to shell out the money for such an expensive flight, but Sarah wisely said, "Pay for a flight now . . . or pay a lot more when you move there and it doesn't work out." She also reminded me of how good it was at UNR, with Ms. King looking after all of her Hughesians. Her advice was timely inasmuch as Sarah herself transferred schools, moving to Las Vegas to be with her boyfriend, and she had faced the same situation.

Albert and I flew to South Carolina together while Mom looked after Jonathan, and his family was exactly as he had portrayed them to me. They were exceedingly friendly, and his mother greeted me with a warm smile.

"Where's that Jonathan?" she asked. "I can't wait to hug him."

I explained that we hadn't brought him, but maybe she would get a chance to see him next time, although I was far from certain that there would ever *be* a next time. Albert's extended family was made up of good people who lived a simple, no frills existence, embracing me as I was introduced to each member.

I tried not to be judgmental, but from the first moments I encountered them and surveyed their property—the trailers and the farmyard animals—I couldn't imagine living there. Albert was totally at ease now that he was back with his folks, but I instinctively knew I would feel isolated from the more sophisticated friends and living conditions I'd grown accustomed to for most of my life.

"You want chicken for lunch?" Albert's mother asked. "You must be hungry from traveling so far."

"Yes, please," I said. "That sounds nice."

She left to prepare a meal while I made small talk with Albert's family, and small talk was probably the right word for it. Their conversation centered around people in the local community and their favorite television shows. Their back and forth was about *their* life, which I couldn't really relate to. When I offered an occasional remark out of politeness, they looked at me like I was speaking a foreign language. My language, in a very real sense, was that of Organic Chemistry, history, microbiology, and all of the events that made up campus life and the various pre-requisites for attending medical school. Although my family had never been rich, I was essentially a gifted student with an intellectual bent, a city girl, pure and simple. Despite their warmth, I felt nothing in common with them.

Later, Albert's mother emerged with lunch, which consisted of southern soul food, such as black-eyed peas and collard greens. "And we have fresh chicken!" she exclaimed happily.

I wondered what made chickens fresh other than the freezer case at the supermarket. I suddenly knew what Albert's mother was getting at as he picked up a wing. "Fresh" meant the chickens out back. The family laughed at me good-naturedly, but I just smiled as I picked up a drumstick. I could handle their teasing with no problem, but as I ate it, I pictured Albert's mother running around the yard feverishly to catch a chicken, grabbing its neck, putting it on a tree stump, and whacking its head with an axe. I thought I'd just as soon eat chicken from the grocery store.

* * *

The visit had given me my answer, and once back in Reno I explained to Albert as gently as possible that the relationship wasn't going to work. Over and above the obvious differences in our education and cultural backgrounds, I had invested too much time at UNR—Ms King, as usual, was right on the money—and Jonathan was now established in daycare and speech therapy, and another move wouldn't be in his best interest. My mother had always said, "Never end a relationship worse off than you were before it began," and the words rang true. My relationship with Albert had given me hope that someone would find me desirable and would also treat Jonathan with kindness. The break-up would also free Albert to be with someone who really wanted to be with him and who appreciated his lifestyle. He would be a great husband for somebody—somebody who wanted a family right away—but not for me. Albert was greatly saddened by my reasoning, but didn't try to contest my decision. Even as we went our own ways, he remained an understanding man who respected me—and accepted me for who I was. It was a bittersweet time of my life, for I had already bought him slippers for Father's Day. I was sad because he would have been a great father for Jonathan.

But I still had my son. He put his arms around my neck and climbed on me. It was fun to play with him, even if it was only just us.

* * *

18

In the Fall of 1996 I was proud to have survived a year of Organic Chemistry, with an overall GPA of 3.7. I hoped my junior year would be even better since the Nevada Women's Fund continued to grant me scholarships. Things were going well enough, in fact, so that I could buy Mom's Ford Escort since she was purchasing a new car for her fiftieth birthday. I now had wheels of my own!

I made additional money as a student coordinator for a summer science minority program for Reno and Las Vegas high school students, much like the programs I myself had attended. It was a positive experience inasmuch as the students' enthusiasm for careers in health and science inspired me to keep moving forward towards my own goals.

One problem that was vexing, however, was my loneliness, and the fact that weighing 220 pounds might affect whether or not anyone would ever be attracted to me again. I was also worried that my weight might skew the perceptions of doctors and professors when it was time for me to interview for medical school. If they didn't think I was capable of living a healthy life, why should they admit me to a profession that had, as a goal, health and well-being? I decided to go for twenty minute walks every day while pushing Jonathan in his stroller. During one of these walks, the wheel popped off the stroller, but I kept walking. In retrospect, this one episode could serve as a metaphor for my entire life's journey. I wanted to give myself the best shot possible at a relationship, at getting into medical school, and at life in general. The wheels in my life had come off many times, but I had always continued on, no matter how bumpy the ride.

I decided to join the Alpha Epsilon Delta pre-med honor society at the university. Not for the first time, I felt judged when I showed up with Jonathan. I imagined the thoughts of the other students: *Does she really think she's going to get into medical school?* I decided to pay my dues for the sake of my resume, but I quit attending society meetings, opting instead to start my own chapter of the Minority Association of Pre-Health Students. I was the president, and any students who chose to attend would have to accept Jonathan's presence.

The group was open to everyone who was serious about getting into professional schools—nursing, graduate, dental, or medical—but we were less pretentious than Alpha Epsilon Delta, choosing a relaxed atmosphere over the honor society's stricter codes. A few white classmates joined, if only to add diversity to their resume. Cameron, for example, was a tall, white, lanky pre-med student, and we both joked about what interviewers might ask him regarding his participation in our group. Over and above the friendly atmosphere and diversity, I felt that it was indeed important for white students to see minority professionals, just as it was good for minority students, too, to see them.

* * *

After a developmental evaluation, it was determined that Jonathan's speech was delayed. For whatever reason, he was simply behind other students in his age group. He started speech therapy at the Special Children's Clinic, where a speech pathologist advised me that Jonathan might develop learning disabilities as he got older—or might be perfectly normal. The thought of him lagging behind in school was very disconcerting. When he had tantrums, I wondered whether they were just an expression of the terrible twos or his inability to communicate. The clinic's staff taught me a few signs to facilitate communication, but my mother's words still haunted me, namely that I had been at least partially responsible for the disability by not reading to Jonathan enough since I'd been so absorbed in my studies. His behavior was especially frustrating at times, as when he'd open and close the refrigerator constantly, turn the fan on and off, or flush the toilet repeatedly. Even more frustrating were the times when he called me "teacher" instead of "mommy." Was parenting ever going to get easier? Did he know who I was?

* * *

When Aunt Bertha visited me and Mom in October, I was worried that she might be harboring a grudge against me. Over lunch, Aunt B and Mom carried the conversation while I fed macaroni and fish sticks to Jonathan. I wondered how life would have turned out if I had given Jonathan to my aunt. I wouldn't have married Darryl, but would I still be in Reno? I let these thoughts drift through my mind in stream of consciousness fashion as Aunt Bertha asked if we wanted dessert. She was being sweet and kind, taking us to Lane Bryant at the mall after lunch. Without the issue of adoption hanging over our heads, I knew she was being sincere.

Back in the car, I expressed what I had been feeling all during lunch. "Aunt Bertha, I'm sorry for everything. I feel terrible about what happened." My sentiment was heartfelt, for who knew what my aunt had felt when I had taken away her dream?

Her reply took me by surprise. "Baby, don't you know that God is good! All things work for the good for those that love the Lord, child." She smiled. "Don't worry about a thing. I've been blessed."

This reassurance lifted a huge weight from my shoulders. My aunt then asked me about my studies, and I filled her in on my junior year thus far. She seemed proud of me, and I was grateful to have her back in my life.

Aunt B inspired me to attend church regularly, and I became a member of a non-denominational church, the Greater Light Christian Light center. The center was a "come as you are" type of congregation—very informal. Jonathan was welcome, and people were down to earth. Reno is not known for its cultural diversity, but Pastor Taylor was a joyful, overweight African-American family man who connected with his parishioners. He would call people out and prophesy over them, and he often did this to me, saying "Melanie! Stand up!" His words always hit the mark, and I was very glad to have the unconditional support of this very unique church.

* * *

Junior year is the most challenging for pre-med students since that is the year they must take the MCAT, or Medical College Admissions Test, which is a grueling day-long exam on biology, physics, chemistry, and English. MCAT preparation courses are virtually mandatory, although the costs for these sessions are high. The one I was interested in attending cost $895, representing a lot of babysitting and work-study hours. Fortunately, Alice Arndt contributed $600, while Pastor Taylor passed the collection plate, which supplied an additional $300—just the amount I needed, with five dollars to spare.

I continued to do volunteer work to enhance my resume for medical school applications, and put in time with the Salvation Army Clinic. I was amazed at how much could be learned from simple urinalysis, such as the presence of dehydration, drug use, diabetes, and much more. It was time well spent, but I still had nagging questions running through my mind: What if I don't get into med school? Was I wasting my time? In the words of Pastor Taylor, I decided to leave it in the hands of God while doing the footwork. I would control what I could and give med school my best shot.

* * *

My babysitting job posed a great challenge. Jonathan was often cranky, and I didn't get much studying done during my hours on the job. Compounding the problem was that Jonathan and the child I was babysitting, Kenny, kept pushing each other, plus they always had runny noses and were constantly trading colds. It was a noisy and aggravating job, and Kenny's parents could not resist the temptation to compare their little darling to Jonathan. "We can't understand what he's saying," they often remarked. Other times, they would comment on the fact that Kenny was so far ahead of Jonathan in potty training. Kenny's father was particularly hard to stomach with his laidback approach, saying, "Kids will be kids." It was easy for him to mouth such glib aphorisms since his child was at a normal stage of development. It was obvious that he believed that he'd been blessed with "the perfect child." There seemed to be implied criticism that something was wrong with both Jonathan and me because he was lagging behind in certain developmental areas. When Jonathan would have a temper tantrum or start to throw things, I sometimes wondered if giving him to Aunt Bertha would have been the better part of wisdom. In December, Kenny's parents gave us gifts—a remote controlled car and a $25 gift card—but I knew by then that I couldn't continue the job anymore. It was too chaotic.

* * *

It was time to start thinking seriously of what I would include in my application to medical school. Ms. King was my "go to" person when it came to both personal and academic matters. I was concerned that mentioning Jonathan in my application might represent a red flag to an admissions committee. Would they believe that a single mom had what it took to endure the rigorous schedule of medical school and residency?

"Jonathan is a big part of who you are," Ms. King said. "If they don't think the fact that you have pulled all of this off as a young single mother is amazing, then that school may not be the right one for you. Be proud of what you have accomplished."

I agreed with what Ms. King said, but this was the real world. I had learned over the course of almost four years that many people regarded a young single mother as a stigma. There was an option at my disposal, however, to enhance both my pocketbook and resume. I could apply for a national *USA Today* scholarship. This would help financially since I was only receiving $85 a month in child support, money garnered from Darryl's wages. The odds of winning were low because of the intense competition, but I had beaten the odds before. If I failed, it wouldn't be for lack of trying.

In applying for the *USA Today* scholarship, as well as many others, I received letters of recommendation from Doctors Gubanich and Mead—and, of course, Ms. King. I also wrote about my challenges as a Health Sciences pre-med major and my role as a mother. I included that I was extremely involved in research and community service, even speaking at conferences.

The *USA Today* scholarship was especially intriguing, even though it seemed as if getting one was like winning the Lottery since the competition was nationwide. I decided to give myself an edge, however, by studying the applications from past winners. Awardees were profiled in the Life section of the paper, so I examined the winners carefully on microfiche at the library. As I sat down to write my story for the application, I included many details of my life with Jonathan since I had worked so hard to create a better life for both of us. Surely that counted for something in a career that sought wellness and self-improvement.

As was the case so often in my life, I beat the odds. Many weeks later, I received a letter that said, "Congratulations! You have been selected as one of the top 20 *USA Today* college academic team." I read the letter twice, feeling that I had to be dreaming. I had actually pulled it off.

The letter indicated that I was to meet with a local photographer so as to be included in their newspaper. It was also very specific that I bring Jonathan to the photo session since he was a major part of my story. Following Ms. King's advice, as well as my own intuition, my forthrightness about being a single mother had scored big points with the committee. Finally, the letter stated that I and the other awardees would be flown to *USA Today* headquarters in Washington, D.C. for the awards ceremony.

A few weeks later I received a call at four in the morning from a staffer at *USA Today*. I was already awake, getting ready to go to the airport.

"You should go to your nearest local newsstand," she said, "because there is a beautiful photo of a young woman and her son on the front page."

With my hair still in rollers, I threw on a robe, grabbed Jonathan, and went to the 7 Eleven. And there it was—above the fold on the front page (along with stories about O.J. Simpson and the death of Bill Cosby's son) was a picture of me holding Jonathan. I purchased ten copies, telling the cashier excitedly that it was me on page one.

Later that morning, I couldn't help but look at every newsstand I passed in the airport. I felt like a celebrity or a country music star hearing her song on the radio for the first time. On the plane, I flew first class and continued sharing my joyful news, telling the stewardess about my photo on the front page. I was even more overwhelmed when she made an announcement to the passengers.

"Ladies and gentlemen," she said, "I'd like to inform you that we have a celebrity on board. For those of you who have a copy of USA Today, look on the front page and you will see her photograph. She is one of our nation's top college graduates, and she's sitting in seat 1-A."

Everyone clapped and cheered. I had come a long way from my days on a Greyhound bus, when the other passengers drank and played cards near the smelly bathroom in the back.

The ceremony was held at the Mayflower Hotel, which was easily the nicest, most elegant hotel I'd ever visited. When the ceremony was over, I called every relative and friend I had, including Albert, to share my pride and exuberance. The tab for my joy came to $428, but sharing my victory was worth every penny. Alice Arndt was ecstatic and promised to frame the award when I got home so I could proudly display it in my living room.

* * *

I would take another flight a few months later, this time to Los Angeles. *Wheel of Fortune* held auditions for people in Reno, and my friends and I decided to give it a try, so we headed to a local casino where the try-outs were being held. The audition was actually a lot of fun. Trying to show our enthusiasm, a hallmark of all contestants, we got to spin the wheel and take a spelling test, after which we were told that some of us would get a postcard notifying us that we'd been selected and would be flown to southern California. When the postcard arrived three weeks later, I was beginning to feel as if I had the Midas touch. For weeks, I watched the show and tried to solve the puzzles in order to get my mind into "contestant mode." This was my game show homework, along with my regular regimen of biochemistry, anatomy, physiology, and MCAT prep. Jonathan jumped up and down every day, yelling, "Mommy's going to be on TV soon!"

When the time came to appear on the show, Arthur and Linda looked after Jonathan while I was at the studio. I was escorted to a room with the other players—two men—one from New Mexico and the other from Utah. After a few practice rounds to loosen us up, the real taping began.

The year was 1997, when Matt Lauer replaced Bryant Gumbel as co-anchor on the *Today* show. To my amazement, there was a puzzle with his name in it, although the other players didn't seem to have a clue as to who Matt Lauer was, guessing Matt Bauer and Matt Sauer. I always watched *Today* as I got ready for classes each day, so I anxiously waited for my turn. The entire puzzle solution was "Katie Couric and Matt Lauer." For this one bit of knowledge I possessed, I won a staggering $17,000 and was invited for the Friday show, when I won an additional $1000. What a contrast this was for someone who, at one time, had to go to the university pantry to get a box of stale Hamburger Helper.

To celebrate, I took Arthur and Linda to the Cheesecake Factory and laid out $108.89 for our meal. Arthur reached out to take the check, but I pushed his hand away and grabbed it first, saying, "My treat!" This felt so good since I could finally give back to others after so much had been given to me. As Aunt Bertha had said regarding her own life, I felt blessed, as if God were working for the good in all things in my life.

* * *

It was show time. The MCAT was held on campus every spring, and it represented the most important test of any I'd taken thus far in my under-graduate years. The objective was to get double-digit scores in all sections of the test, meaning 10s or higher. Once again I was the fly in the but-termilk, a young African American woman, since so many of my pre-med friends had dropped by the wayside due to the academic difficulty and intensity that came with being a pre-med student. We were given our pencils and test booklets, and I realized that everything came down to this one day. My GPA and community service would count for naught if I blew the MCAT. And then the thought hit me: I had spent so much time study-ing—at times away from Jonathan—in order to get this far. How would I make it through medical school, which would be far more difficult than

my undergrad years? But my religious faith helped to erase these nega-
tive thoughts. I firmly believed that God was making a way for me. He'd
sent me great mentors, helped me with the *USA Today* scholarship, and (I
firmly believed) assisted me in getting onto *Wheel of Fortune*. I was certain
he wanted me to pursue my dream of becoming a doctor.

The weeks following the test were angst-ridden. If my scores were
too low, would I try again in the fall? Would I give up altogether? Time
would tell, but the waiting was excruciating.

* * *

Mom said Darryl had been calling, news that was a far cry from noti-
fications about *USA Today* or the *Wheel of Fortune*. Two years had passed
since I'd seen him, and I wondered where life had taken him. Had he
finally found a healthy path, or maybe even found God? The idea of calling
him was daunting, but I didn't want to be like other mothers, cutting the
biological father out of the picture completely. I owed it to Jonathan to at
least return his call. Swallowing hard, I dialed the number to his mother's
home.

"Hello," said a familiar voice on the other end of the line.

Hearing his voice was eerie, bringing back so many bad memories.

"Hi, Darryl."

"How's my son?" He was blunt as usual.

"He's very happy. He's two now."

I didn't mention Jonathan's tantrums or speech delay. To my way of
thinking, Darryl hadn't earned the right to know details, only generalities
since he hadn't been present for his son's first words even when he'd lived
under the same roof with us.

"Why don't you send me no pictures?"

Darryl had never requested any, so I allowed an awkward silence to
hover over the line. I was frustrated and didn't want to get baited into an
argument.

"You get your money, right?" he said. "Uncle Sam makes damn sure
you get it."

He was alluding to the meager $85 per month in child support. He never sent any clothes, gifts, or Christmas cards to his own son, and the $85 probably wouldn't have arrived every month without the assistance of my lawyer and the government.

"Yes, I get the money. What exactly do you want?" It was a long distance call, and I wanted him to cut to the chase.

"Well, I figured that now that you're rich, you don't need nothing more from me."

I paused and then realized he'd seen me on *Wheel of Fortune*. That's what the call was about, plain and simple.

"Darryl, that money is for Jonathan and me." I was getting defensive and attempted to relate my overall situation to him before realizing that I didn't owe him any explanation at all. I hung up . . . and continued to collect the $85 a month.

It was the last time I would ever hear his voice.

* * *

I began working on my application to the American Medical College Application Service, or AMCAS, which waived application fees to ten schools for low-income students. As I was writing my personal statement and organizing my letters of recommendation, the letter with my MCAT scores arrived.

Too nervous to open the letter myself, I took it to my pre-med advisor and asked her to break the seal and give me the news, good or bad.

"Melanie," she said after an ominous pause, "your scores are mediocre. I wouldn't apply to any top-tier schools if I were you. You'd be wasting your time."

I was crestfallen, my eyes welling up. I sniffled and tried to hold back my tears. The scores were 9, 9 and 7, with not a single double-digit to be seen. I felt as if I was on the verge of hyperventilating as my breath came in rapid bursts. I'd tried my best, but maybe I just wasn't good enough. Indeed, I'd read that students of color often scored lower on standardized tests, so maybe I wasn't as smart as I always assumed myself to be. Maybe

I didn't deserve to go to medical school. My self-esteem plummeted in the space of just a few minutes.

Meanwhile, the other pre-med students were openly talking about their double-digit scores, which further served to enhance my pessimism.

"How'd you do?" asked Tom, a tall white married man in his late twenties. He had two children, was fit, and enjoyed rock climbing. He had support and confidence, and his status as the perfect all-American boy who had it all was something that had intimidated me for several years. His question to me was a bit too challenging.

"Good enough," I replied, caught off guard.

He handed me his scores: 10, 10, and 12.

"That's great, Tom," I said, forcing a smile.

"Where are you applying?" he asked, perhaps sensing my inferiority.

"I'm going to meet with my advisor," I said, not telling him I'd already consulted her. "And I will, of course, be applying here."

I didn't bother to ask him where he was applying. I didn't really want to hear his answer, and I slowly backed away from him, ending the conversation.

I picked up Jonathan at the Y, and he looked happy to see me. I wanted to be happy, too, that day, but it was hard. The King Midas touch seemed to have evaporated.

* * *

My inclination was to play it safe and apply to the University of Nevada Medical School. Even if I managed to get interviews elsewhere despite my mediocre MCAT scores, I would have to spend a lot of money on airfare, hotels, and taxis. I'd also have to coordinate Jonathan's care with my mother.

But I had the *Wheel of Fortune* money coming in, and it seemed that if I settled for a "sure thing" that I would be reliving my TAMS experience. I wanted more out of med school than the basics—the medical equivalent of reading, writing, and 'rithmetic—and I wanted to at least see what the other schools had to offer. There was no harm in applying to the schools since the application fees were waived, so I applied to California schools, where family would be close by and where I had heard that minority students had good support. I therefore sent applications to UCLA, USC, Stanford—all representing short flights with low airfares—and other schools across the country. Nothing ventured, nothing gained.

I was again taking the bulls by the horn and not allowing bad news to deter me from seeking what I truly wanted, but the bull was awfully tough, and I was getting tired. Jonathan turned three a few days later. I bought him a cake and party favors with a *Toy Story* theme. Jonathan fell asleep on his bed without having dinner. I didn't want to wake him, so I climbed into bed with him and decided to rest. I would make a really good breakfast in the morning. That would have to do.

I was worn out.

* * *

I was fortunate enough to be offered interviews at half of the schools to which I'd applied, which included Washington University in St. Louis, St. Louis University, the Mayo Clinic, USC (University of Southern California), and Stanford. My advisor had been wrong, and I wondered how many other students had followed her misguided advice. But now it was time to prepare for the actual trips—there would be several—and to look as professional as possible. The bright pink suit I'd worn on *Wheel of Fortune* wasn't appropriate for such interviews, with navy blazer and skirt being the standard. I decided to wear my hair in a French twist and accent my suit with pearl earrings and necklace, hoping I could buy real ones one day. To top things off, Aunt Bertha sent me a burgundy briefcase. In it I placed a notepad, a novel to distract me, my *USA Today* story, and my optimism.

The interview process was intimidating. I'd purchased books on the interviewing process and how to maintain poise and confidence. A candidate needed to be self-assured but not arrogant, asking pertinent questions. I also kept up on current events, knowing that the questions I might receive could cover any topic a committee member wished to visit. Other students on the interview circuit were intimidating in their own right, students from Duke, Stanford, and Yale. They were calm and seemed as if getting into any medical school was a *fait accompli*. My only strategy was to use what had brought me through so much turmoil: Be myself. I was Melanie Watkins. That's who I was and that's all I needed.

After the many long and sometimes grueling trips—the drive to the Mayo Clinic in Rochester was on a bitter cold day with a bleak landscape stretching for miles in every direction—I was delighted to learn that I was accepted at every school that interviewed me. They were willing to take a chance on a single mother. Still, making a final decision was difficult. Stanford was one of the most respected schools in the country, but it was also one of the most expensive schools in the San Francisco Bay area.

Then the whispers started, accompanied by a cold shoulder from some of my fellow students, both pre-med and others. *The only reason she was accepted to Stanford is because she's black.* Thankfully, Cameron, who'd been with me for long study sessions in the library, was aware of my awards, community service, and volunteer work, and his validations counted for a lot. I didn't doubt that race had played some role in determining whether I had been accepted into the various medical schools or not, but I also thought with dismay about my mediocre test scores. Would I make a good doctor? I was angry, feeling as if I were the "token" used to fill a given school's quota.

I called Tonya to tell her how hurt I was by the gossip circulating among my peers.

"Melanie," she said, "they're just jealous that *they* didn't get accepted into Stanford, too."

I thought about how my sister often teased me for being book smart, but not "street smart," as she was. She had, on several occasions, called me "oreo," meaning that I was white on the inside and black on the outside. Perhaps she herself was jealous of my accomplishments, but it still hurt to hear this from a family member. I felt caught: I wasn't black enough for Tonya, but I wasn't white enough for my pre-med peers. All of these thoughts served to minimize my achievements in my own mind.

But what if they were right? I didn't really believe this—not deep down—but it was a thought that left a bad taste in my mouth after the

Herculean struggles I'd been through to find a career in medicine. Mitigating these unpleasant reflections was the fact that other ethnicities, such as Native Americans and Latinos, had not been accepted at Stanford or other prestigious schools, and some of them had even attended Ivy League colleges. I, on the other hand, was coming from a state university. To Ms. King, that naturally made no difference at all, nor did it make any difference to her that I was being gossiped about or that I had attended UNR. She told me to remember that I was a Hughesian and to get a thick skin—and quickly.

Tom approached me again one day, casually remarking that he'd heard I'd been accepted at Stanford. He still was fishing for my MCAT scores and asked yet again what they were.

"Good enough to get into Stanford," I answered, putting Ms. King's advice into practice in short order.

"You know, Melanie," he said, "those students at Stanford. . . ." He looked down for emphasis and then looked me in the eyes. "Those students are really, really smart."

Was he implying that I wasn't—or that I wasn't up to the challenge?

Ignoring his comment, I asked him which school he had chosen.

"I'm staying here in Reno," he said. "As you know, I have a wife and kids, and we own a house."

"Congratulations," I said before walking away. I wasn't going to stand around and be judged. He had gotten the double-digit scores, but I was the one going to Stanford.

* * *

Mom wanted me to stay in Reno as well. She was enjoying her grandson and also believed that it made sense for me to stay in familiar surroundings, where class sizes were smaller, tuition was less expensive—and where I had family support, which was indeed important.

Stanford, however, was only a four-hour drive from Reno, and it would afford me far more opportunities than UNR. Even better, there was a daycare facility and elementary school on campus. As if that wasn't enough, the university offered family housing on campus, and the area was quite safe given Stanford's prestigious reputation. While I wanted my mother's support and realized that I didn't have any friends in northern California, I wanted to cut the umbilical cord and assert my independence. Being conflicted, I asked many of my friends for their opinions, including the medical student and his wife, Stacey and Samantha, who had been so supportive when I'd lived at Stead. Stacey had definite opinions on the matter. "Research schools are just that," he said. "Schools like that can be very traditional, hierarchical, and competitive. You won't get to talk to the attendings who teach the med students and residents, plus it's very expensive, Melanie."

I appreciated his candor, but I remained undecided. Later that week, I made an appointment with Dr. Thornton, my ethics professor, figuring that if anyone could sift through the different variables that had to be dealt with in making an important decision, it would be someone grounded in the field of ethics. She was an elderly lady with graying blond hair, round glasses, and modest jewelry. Surprisingly, her answer to my questions was a personal story.

"When I was your age," she began, "I wanted to become a lawyer. So did my husband. We were both accepted at Stanford, but because we had two young sons—" She paused, choking up slightly. "Well, I made the decision to raise our sons. I continued to think about going to law school, but ultimately, I opted for graduate school instead. That was twenty-five years ago," she said wistfully. "If I had the opportunity to attend Stanford again. . . ." She paused a second time. "Go to Stanford, Melanie. It's not a chance you'll ever have again. If you stay in Reno, you may always have regrets—always have the "what if" lingering in your thoughts."

This advice wasn't the balanced answer I'd expected, but it was heartfelt and direct, and for that reason, perhaps more valuable.

"But it's so expensive," I countered. "I can't afford it."

"I will help you."

I didn't know what she meant at the time, but months later, as Jon and I packed the Ford Escort with luggage while my friend Marge helped me load her pick-up truck before we caravanned to the campus at Palo Alto, I checked my mailbox one last time and found a letter from Dr. Thornton. As it turned out, her husband wasn't just any lawyer, but a very important and affluent one. "Melanie," the letter read, "I want to support you and Jonathan. I will pay for his childcare while you're at Stanford. Send me the bill every month, and I'll send you a check. Good luck to you and Jonathan!"

I clutched the letter to my chest and then picked up Jonathan and whirled him in circles.

"We're on our way, Jonathan!" I cried. "We're on our way!"

As Pastor Taylor had said, I'd done the footwork, and God had executed his plan for my life thus far. He had indeed worked for the good in all things in my life, even when I couldn't see his hand during my pain and blindness. My summers outside of Shreveport, listening to my grandparents speak of the Lord, had not been wasted.

* * *

19

Heading up University Drive at Stanford, lined with stately California palms, is an awe-inspiring experience when one considers that this beautiful lane leads to one of the greatest learning centers in the world. I had paid a heavy price to earn the right to drive onto campus as a student, coming a long way from the streets of Jackson, Mississippi, where a young woman of color had battled just to graduate from high school. But *every* path I'd traveled—the metaphorical ones such as marriage and college, as well as the real ones on airplanes and Greyhound buses—had led me to Stanford, where it was now time to begin traveling the most important path yet: the one that would lead to my becoming a physician. I desperately wanted to help others, especially young women who had faced the very same trials I had.

Medical school is usually divided into two sections. The first two years are the pre-clinical years, which, through lab work and study, lay the foundation for later training. Year one emphasizes the study of anatomy, histology, and embryology, while year two is devoted to pathology, or the study how diseases progress—and why. The last two years of training ease students into actually seeing patients under the supervision of attending physicians as they make rounds and assign various duties to their "understudies," such as taking case histories or researching various diseases and their underlying pathologies.

Beyond this traditional partition of phases within medical schools, Stanford offers their students the choice of a traditional four-year curriculum beyond or an extended educational experience allowing them to study other, more diverse courses in five or six-year programs that afford them the opportunity to travel and obtain valuable clinical experience in a variety of settings. I had chosen my university wisely.

But when a student graduates from medical school, this does not represent the end of training by any means, even though one has earned the right to put the initials M.D. behind his or her name. Students must advance to internship, residency, and at times a fellowship. Also, some specialties call for a longer residency than others. Some students wish to follow in the footsteps of a family member (e.g. becoming neuro-, cardio-, or vascular surgeons), but I wanted to specialize in obstetrics/gynecology, even though it was a long and difficult residency. I wanted to help teen mothers, sharing with them my own experiences, encouraging them to pursue their dreams and not settle for a lackluster existence that awaited TAMS graduates. I envisioned myself making rounds and delivering babies. In my own small way, I would become to them what Ms. King had been to me.

It would also be an excellent way of giving a portion of my life to God after all he had given to me.

* * *

Our class of eighty-six nervous students gathered in a lecture hall at the beginning of the semester as Dr. Mathers, our anatomy professor, stood at the podium. He had a slight paunch hanging over his belt, but it wasn't so big that he wasn't able to tuck in his shirt. A fifty-something with both an M.D. and a PhD, he looked out over the sea of faces and made a surprising statement to start our medical careers: "Welcome 1998 incoming class. Today, I am happy to say, I have finally paid off my student loans."

We didn't know whether to laugh or not until he himself laughed a few seconds later. But was he telling the truth? Were we embarking on a road of unimagineable debt? I was receiving a great deal of scholarship money and private assistance (through Ms. Arndt and Dr. Thornton), but how many years would I have to face financial hardship?

I was surprised that not all of my classmates were in their early to mid-twenties. Some were in their thirties and forties—accountants, lawyers, engineers, teachers, and other professionals. This diverse group seemed dynamic and bright, and I recalled Tom's comment about how smart Stanford students were. Maybe he'd been right when giving me his subtle cues about my ability to compete. My thoughts were interrupted by Dr. Mather's next remarks as he dove effortlessly into his lecture with the ease of a professor who had taught for years.

"You will be placed in groups of four, and each group will be assigned to a cadaver. You should also be familiar with your classmates' cadavers so as to become knowledgeable about both male and female anatomy. But your dissection team will primarily work on just one cadaver."

I'd known that this was going to be an important part of medical school and had had limited experience with cadavers as an undergraduate, when classes had to learn how to identify various organs, tissues, muscles, and tendons. In medical school, however, we ourselves would be doing the dissecting.

"You will have a key to the anatomy room," Dr. Mathers continued, "as well as a case with skeletal bones in order to memorize structures of the body. You can spend as much time as you need with your cadaver."

I couldn't envision myself leaving Jonathan at ten in the night to "spend more time with my cadaver"—a scenario out of Stephen King movie—but I wondered if that was the kind of dedication required to succeed. Would my classmates be in the anatomy lab until the wee hours of the morning?

"You will smell like phenol and formaldehyde," Dr. Mathers explained. "These are the normal chemicals used to preserve tissues. Okay now. Let's walk to the anatomy room."

I wanted to sink down in my seat and not move. We all looked at each other, wondering what we had gotten ourselves into. With trepidation, my friend Karen and I entered the lab, a cold room where the cadavers were stored in zipped black bags. The smell was pungent.

"This is how we're going to smell for the next four years," she whispered. She was confident, but then she'd been at Stanford for college. I was a Hughesian, but was I in the same league as Karen and others?

I looked at the row of bags. Who *were* these people, and what misfortunes had brought them here? In time I would learn that most of the bodies we would dissect were older men and women who had donated their bodies to science. People who died at a younger age usually had their organs harvested for transplant. Sicker individuals, young or old, were not considered viable cadavers since diseases such as cancer might render their organs unidentifiable.

Dr. Mathers disappeared momentarily and came back with his blue scrubs on, which is when the teaching assistants—students who had previously excelled in anatomy—began to unzip the bags. Most of the cadavers were elderly Caucasians, and I noted that one still had nail polish on her fingernails. Another had a relatively new surgical scar. Nearby, a black woman lay cold and forever silent, eyes closed and lips full. I wondered what she had been thinking when she had decided to do this. Could she have foreseen such a moment even though she wanted medical students to gain valuable knowledge from her body? Would she still have consented if she could have somehow magically seen what was about to happen to her lifeless body? I was glad to have been assigned to a thin white elderly male. The African American woman looked as if she could have been a family member, and working on her would have hit much too close to home. I looked away from the nearest row of zipped bags.

"Let's take a moment of silence, gratitude, and acknowledgement," Dr. Mathers said, an allusion to the selflessness of those who had donated their bodies.

Swallowing hard, I allowed myself to look at the cadavers again.

"Thank you," I whispered to God, my own prayer of thanksgiving for being allowed to start my medical career in earnest.

* * *

My headaches returned that September. The migraines hit almost every day, and I recall Jonathan, whose speech had improved to the point where he could say "headache," touching my forehead as I lay in the dark while he watched *Dumbo* on TV. I tried reciting he twenty-third psalm over and over—*The Lord is my shepherd, I shall not want*—in order to alleviate the pain. My appetite was gone because of the nausea, a very minor blessing since I had gained the twenty pounds I'd lost in my senior year. Eating had become my way of dealing with stress. The pain was so excruciating at times that I would revisit all of my decisions—should I have given Jonathan to Aunt B, stayed with Albert, or gone to school in Reno?

The doctor at the student health center prescribed Elavil and Imitrex for the pain. These meds, along with prayer, helped me through my first semester. The curriculum was a Pass/Fail system (and I would go on to score well enough in all my classes to pass), although medical school was every bit as difficult as I'd expected. It was just a matter of time, I feared, before the migraines returned again.

* * *

Jonathan and I secured very nice housing—town house style again—in an area called Escondido Village. Jonathan attended a pre-school in the morning (just a short bike ride away, which meant no more bus rides), and daycare in the afternoon. Indeed, biking was the primary means of transportation on campus, and Mrs. Arndt had continued to supply Jonathan with wonderful gifts from his wish list, such as new bikes when necessary. The village was an "instant community." Several wives of grad students performed babysitting chores, and I responded in kind whenever possible, although they had far more time than I did. Despite the pleasant atmosphere of the community, I knew that I'd eventually need more help since studying three to four hours per night was the norm. Every week was like preparing for final exams.

As for my classmates, they were an interesting, motivated bunch that accepted Jonathan immediately. They often came over to my apartment—a stark contrast to the horror I experienced in Stead, where I was ashamed for my friends to see Darryl's trash and empty beer cans—and we would watch ER, picking up terms such as "CBC," "ABG," or "chem panel." It was easy for me to imagine using these phrases one day in a hospital as nurses and other staff carried out my orders.

Jonathan was making the adjustment to campus life quite nicely, and he always wrapped his arms around me and gave me a big kiss no matter what I smelled like after long, tough days of studying anatomy. He even had a spunky four-year-old girlfriend named Madison who informed me that one day she would most definitely marry my son. As for me, I was older now and was accepted as Jon's mother, which suited me just fine. The stigma of single "teen mother" was finally gone.

That didn't mean I wasn't lonely. I was jealous of other students who could take time off to party, for with no children to tie them down, they could escape to San Francisco, only forty-five minutes away. I wasn't invited to many of these outings because my friends assumed correctly that I wouldn't be able to go. I also feared that they might be embarrassed by my weight in a social setting, but I had no outlet to deal with stress. Sensing this, Karen told me that her little sister Brianna was coming to town and asked me if I wanted to join them on their trip into the city the following Friday.

"Come on, Melanie," she said. "You need to get out and have a little fun."

This was just what I needed. I asked Madison's mom to look after Jonathan, and so I was set to have a little fun for the first time in a long while. On Friday, Karen, Brianna, and I headed for the San Francisco. Brianna seemed young an immature, rolling her eyes as Karen and I vented about medical school.

Waiting in a long line outside the club, I wondered if I would meet somebody. I wasn't looking for a long-term relationship, just somebody to date and hang out with, assuming anyone found me attractive to begin with. The last time I'd slept with anyone, he'd wet the bed! I craved intimacy and attention, but in the meantime, I just wanted to dance and let off some steam.

We made it to the front of the line and presented our identification to the bouncer, who looked at Brianna's ID, then at Brianna, then back at the ID.

"This won't work," he said, flicking aside the ID card.

"What?" asked Brianna.

"Nope," he reiterated. "Doesn't fly."

Crestfallen, we stepped aside.

Brianna shrugged her shoulders, saying in a cavalier manner, "Whatever. I've never had any problems with the card before." She shrugged as walked back to the car.

I was fuming. I'd gone through a great deal of effort to secure a babysitter, dress, prepare for the evening, drive an hour, find parking, and it had all been for nothing. Karen should have told me up front that her sister was underage. If nothing else, I could have used the precious time to study. Karen saw the look I gave her sister and said, "Aw, Mel just wanted to go to the club." I resented both of them, however, since they didn't have children and could try again the next night. I couldn't. Maybe I really was an overweight woman they'd brought out of pity.

I desperately needed to find an outlet for my frustration. Deciding that maybe my priorities were skewed, I took Jonathan to the AME, or African Methodist Episcopalean church in Palo Alto and sat in the back since I wasn't sure Jon could make it through a ninety-minute service. A quick exit might have been needed.

Pastor Harrison was a younger version of Pastor Taylor, preaching with passion. I needed a church family, and I was pleased when Jonathan clapped to the music, his legs swinging to and fro beneath the pew. This needed to be his family as much as mine. After the service, I met the pastor as we walked through the door.

"Welcome to our congregation" Pastor Harrison said, "and thank you for both coming today!" He looked down at Jonathan, who instinctively said, "Thank you."

I went home feeling good about my new family. My renewed faith also reminded me that I'd neglected my journal writing as well, so I resumed recording my thoughts as time permitted, and it proved to be a great source of stress relief.

I wanted to give my brain a break by reading something non-medical, so I read *Chicken Soup for the Woman's Soul*, a book given to me by Marge (who was an older student going for a PhD in nutrition sciences). I enjoyed the format of the book, which contained thoughtful and inspiring stories that one could read in five minutes or less. Given my long history of journal writing, I decided I would like to write a similar piece since the back pages had instructions on how to submit a story. "Let's write a story together," I told Jonathan, heading to the computer room in our town house. Once there, I wrote a brief account of being a single mother negotiating her first year of medical school. Regardless of the outcome, I felt it to have been an enjoyable experience for both Jon and me. It was a simple piece, written quickly but sincerely.

The King Midas Touch returned, for a few months later, I received a letter notifying me that the story was going to be published in *Chicken Soup for the Single's Soul*. Additionally, it was slated to appear in *Women's World* magazine. It was the pick-me up that I needed. The first semester of medical school had been like taking five O-Chem classes all at once, and I wondered if I would remember half of what I'd learned. Still, the publication of my story reminded me that a greater force was moving behind the scenes to help me along. King Midas was, in actuality, my Father in heaven.

* * *

20

Dr. Matthews, an African-American psychiatrist, had interviewed me when I was applying to Stanford. In his mid-fifties and dressed in natty bow tie, he had a way of putting me at ease, so that our time together seemed more like a therapy session than an interview.

"Melanie," he said, "tell me why you want to become a doctor."

"To help people," I said, "and because I've always liked science. It seems like a logical field for me."

He leaned back in his chair and repeated the question. "Melanie, tell me why you want to become a doctor."

I wanted to be very professional in my responses, but his probing question was beginning to penetrate a very personal part of my life. I wasn't sure how to provide a cogent answer that covered my emotions rather than logical decision-making.

"Because I need to," I said. "I want to be the kind of doctor that people such as me need to have. I need the opportunity to make a difference in people's lives, and that includes my own life and my son Jonathan's."

I was speaking from the heart, and I hoped my words resonated with Dr. Matthews.

From that single interview months earlier, I felt that Dr. Matthews knew more about me than any other faculty member on campus. He called me in periodically to check on me and, working with other faculty members of color at the medical school, made sure that I was adjusting to campus life and the rigors of being a med student. Like Ms. King before him, he quickly became a mentor and role model. He and his wife were both African American psychiatrists, and they had an only child who was

Jonathan's age. I wondered if I, too, might someday have both a professional life and marriage such as theirs.

He called one evening to ask how I was doing. He already knew the answer, of course, which was that I was swamped with work and overwhelmed like all of the other students right before finals.

"Hanging in there," I said, trying to sound upbeat.

"My family and I are going to Lake Tahoe this weekend to go skiing and . . ."

I zoned out completely, instantly jealous of family vacations. Surely he wasn't inviting me, knowing that final exams were around the corner, nor could I have afforded such a getaway at *any* time of the semester. Vacations? I'd spent my summers near Shreveport, but as a rule, vacations had never been a part of my family's budget.

". . . and we would like to take Jonathan with us so you can have more time to study for finals. If that's all right with you, of course."

All right? Of course is was all right! A huge weight had been lifted from my shoulders by yet another person God had set in my path, someone with a heart big enough to make such a magnanimous gesture. Jonathan had never been skiing, and I imagined how cute he would look in a little ski outfit while playing in the snow. I would naturally miss him, but in a very real sense, my time studying was for both of us. My success in medical school would ultimately be his success as well.

* * *

My classmates had been the best and brightest at their various undergrad institutions, but regrettably some failed anatomy, and it was a harsh blow for those who did. I, however, made it through, saving me from more agonizing doubts about whether or not I was worthy of being called Dr. Watkins. My self-esteem was also intact thanks to the feedback from my story. After the *Chicken Soup* story was published, I received emails from males, females, parents, adults, and children, all of which I printed out and posted to the wall of my bedroom. Even Dr. Mathers sent me a congratulatory email with "Your Chicken Soup" in the subject line, giving me praise for being a single mom successfully coping with med school. Furthermore, things eased financially when I sublet a room to another first-year medical student, who proved to be a valuable study partner.

Jonathan and I shared a room at this time, but my study partner intended to move out the following semester in order to live with his girlfriend. With Jonathan back from Tahoe, I knew I was going to need help when the second semester began since he would usually wait up for me until I'd finished studying for the evening. At times, I would have to lie down with him at 8 p.m., sneaking away to the living room to study, hoping he wouldn't discover my absence. Karen suggested I get a nanny, informing me that this was how many moms in the Palo Alto area managed a family while holding down a job. The idea sounded great in theory, but I knew I would have to take out additional loans to find a nanny. Many in the profession wanted their employers to provide health-care insurance, money to use toward education, travel expenses, their own car, and room and board. It occurred to me that I might have done better financially by becoming a nanny instead of enrolling in graduate school.

What I needed was someone to be at home with Jonathan when I needed to attend study sessions, someone who was kind, honest, outgoing, and responsible, but I could only offer room and board in exchange for childcare. I placed an ad in the Stanford campus newspaper and scheduled interviews. I spoke with grandmotherly types as well as students, but all applicants had other constraints that restricted the hours they could work in the evenings or on weekends. Just when I thought that the idea wasn't going to pan out, the phone rang.

"I'm interested in the nanny position," stated a male voice.

The man was honest in telling me that he didn't actually have formal experience in being a nanny, but he said he liked kids and would be available most evenings and weekends. He had great references, an MBA, and was interested in working on a start-up company using manpower drawn from Stanford undergraduates. All he needed was a room to use a base of operations in his spare time. My gut told me this was the right person, so I asked him to stop by on a Saturday afternoon. When I answered the door,

I could hardly believe my eyes. He was six-two, had blue eyes and dark brown hair, and flashed an All-American smile.

"Hi," he said, extending his hand. "I'm Mark."

I took his hand, trying not to stare at him. He was quite handsome.

Mark laughed and appeared unfazed when Jonathan tried to climb all over him and pull his cap. Within the first ten minutes of his arrival, Mark and Jonathan were already playing as I explained what the position would entail. There seemed to be an instant bond between the two. I told him we would love to have him as our nanny, but not before running a question by him that I hadn't foreseen asking any candidate: "Are you single?"

* * *

I wasn't required to see any patients yet—that was for my clinical years on the wards—but we did have to take An Introduction to Clinical Medicine, which would give us an opportunity to practice our interviewing skills. We were given questionnaires inserted within a laminated template that could be attached to a clipboard. The questions sought to gain information about various organ systems through inquiries such as "Do you cough, sneeze, have seasonal allergies, or hay fever?" By far the most challenging section of the questionnaire dealt with the genitourinary system since it entailed questions about incontinence, dribbling, and sexually transmitted behavior. We got the chance to observe each other conducting such interviews, although the interviewees were paid actors pretending to be patients. It was nevertheless going to be nerve-wracking since I had to ask numerous questions—"Do you wear seatbelts, own a firearm, or have ever been the victim of domestic violence?"—within a one-hour timeframe.

I put on my white coat and headed toward the interview room. All interviews were taped so that incoming med students could evaluate their performances, although I sensed I wouldn't be showing my particular tape to people with the same pride as when I'd played back my *Wheel of Fortune* appearance. We didn't know who would be chosen first, so we all remained a bit apprehensive.

Brian, one of my anatomy partners, got the nod. Blond, blue-eyed, and sharp, he'd made it clear from the beginning of the semester that he wanted to become a neurosurgeon. He was therefore one of the students who did indeed spend time in the cadaver room late at night, going the extra mile because of the intricacies of his expected specialty. Being in a room full of dead people, however, didn't require any developed social skills. Talking to a live patient would be different.

Despite Brian's great intelligence, he was awkward in his interviewing skills. Barely making eye contact with his patient, he stared at his clipboard while asking the list of questions in a rote manner. He was talking fast, flying through the inquiries on respiratory, cardiovascular, and neurological systems. The real challenge came when he had to ask his sixty-two-year old married, male Caucasian patient about the genitourinary system. Without missing a beat, he said, "So tell me Mr. Weller, do you have sex with men, women, or both?"

"Just my wife," the man replied, clearing his throat. "We've been married forty years."

"Okay," Brain said. "Married. Fine. Umm, is it hard to get all the urine out when you go to the bathroom?"

We cringed in horror while Brian continued, wiping away perspiration falling on his clipboard as he queried the man about penile discharge, erectile dysfunction, and premature ejaculation. We were all relieved when it was over.

Well, not quite. We would all have to take our turn in the course of the semester. Fortunately, we were able to watch our instructor conduct an interview on tape as he allowed topics to flow seamlessly from one to the other. Even with limited time, he didn't seem rushed. As a doctor, his clinical skills were sharp, but it sometimes felt to the rest of us that we were just pretending to be doctors, much like the actors pretending to be patients.

For every mile I traveled, my path seemed to extend that much farther into the distance.

* * *

Mark was a tremendous help to me during the second part of the year, and I was especially enthusiastic about the presence of Jonathan having a male role model in his life. This had been an issue I'd been concerned about for a very long time. Mark didn't represent a perfect solution (even though I was often mesmerized by his looks), but for now it was a win-win situation. I had help, and Jonathan had a great guy to look up to.

That didn't mean I was at ease and coasting through my first year. Because of the stress of school, I was gaining weight again. Even the scrubs were too tight, and I was wearing XL clothes. I felt fatigued all the time and forced myself to exercise, hoping it would lift my mood. On the western side of the campus is an area simply known as "the dish," where a satellite dish is located and where students and faculty like to hike. I decided to take Jonathan with me one morning and attempt to trek up the steep incline leading to the dish, but I struggled with every step. It was discouraging to see a jogger zooming right past me as if were expending no effort at all. Jon and I continued on, but I had to pause every few minutes, out of breath and sweating. Even an elderly Asian couple passed us, and I could only stare at them in disbelief. How could I have gotten so out of shape while being so busy all the time?

"Mommy, pick me up!" pleaded Jonathan.

I looked at how far we had come on the trail—and how far we still had to go. I just stopped. Jonathan was tugging at my sweatpants, but I didn't feel like I had the energy to continue. I was stuck. Jonathan and I sat down on the side of the trail and watched hikers going up the incline.

"Look, Mommy!" he cried, spying a lizard sunning itself on a rock.

"Oh," I replied rather listlessly.

I wanted to display excitement at his discovery, but the truth was that I wasn't finding joy in anything. No matter how many hours of sleep I got each night, it was never enough. Everyone else in my life seemed so happy. Like the hikers on the trail, the busy world kept moving, and, likewise, my friends were going on with their lives despite the stress of medical school. I was feeling left behind.

We eventually descended the trail, but in time I started to experience suicidal thoughts. Due to my religious background and having to care for

Jonathan, the thoughts were fleeting, but I was afraid of living alone—even dying alone. Who would take care of Jonathan if something happened to me? My mind was in a very dark place.

I'd had too many triumphs not to push forward, so I made an appointment at the student health clinic. Maybe I had an under-active thyroid gland or was anemic? Or perhaps even cancer since that, too, can cause fatigue. Like a lot of medical students, I ran through every disease that I had studied, wondering if my symptoms fit.

The nurse practitioner at the clinic talked with me about my symptoms. I had difficulty concentrating, was sad and tearful, had no energy, was irritable, and wanted to stay in bed and sleep most of the time. Everything seemed like such an effort, and I didn't even want to play with Jonathan anymore.

"I'm sending you to the lab for blood work," the nurse said, "so that we can rule out everything, but it appears you're suffering from depression. It's not surprising since you are under tremendous stress and have a family history of mental illness."

This was a reference to the information I'd provided regarding my family on the routine check-in forms. My uncle Johnny had suffered from schizophrenia. He'd disappeared when I was eight. Aunt Linda had bipolar disorder and was living in a group home in Tennessee, where she'd ended up after taking a Greyhound to the state and publicly disrobing. My cousin Kathy had been a high school valedictorian, but she had a psychotic break when she went to college. She'd dropped out of school and had been living at home ever since.

Was it possible that medical school was driving me crazy? Could it make me psychotic, like Kathy? No, I knew I was in touch with reality, but perhaps the real delusion was that I could make it through college as a single mom. I'd endured a lot of stress in my life, but maybe this was the proverbial end of the line. Maybe it was time to adopt more realistic expectations.

Tonya, who was pregnant with her second child and was continuing in her role as a single working mother, had already sensed that I was depressed. We laughed together, thinking how black women don't have time to be depressed. Depression was one disease reserved for white people. They could afford that luxury. We couldn't.

Or so I thought.

"I'm referring you to the psychiatric clinic," the nurse said. "There are residents there who can provide therapy."

I thought back to when a college psych grad had told me to eat well, get enough sleep, and exercise. What kind of help could I get from additional generalities and platitudes?

"And here's a prescription for Prozac, 20mg daily," she said, handing me the script.

"Do I really need medicine?"

She nodded. "If you have heart disease or a broken ankle, you take the appropriate medication, right?"

She had a point, especially in light of the fact that I was in training to do just was she herself was doing at that very moment. I started to cry, realizing that I couldn't handle one more stressor. I had Jonathan to take care of, I was getting migraines, I was overweight, and I had to use every spare minute I could squeeze from my daily schedule for studying. And it was going to take time to make and keep my appointments. I felt as if I had a hundred things on my "to do" list. I had a full plate, and the nurse had just dished out "get treatment for depression" on top of everything else.

It took tremendous effort just to leave the clinic and walk to my bike, but I needed to pick up Jonathan at daycare. I'd fill the prescription—when I had the time.

* * *

I stared at the bottle, feeling conflicted. I wanted to get better—*needed* to get better—but in my depressed state, I was thinking "Why bother? It's just a pill."

I called Albert since we had reached a point where we could reminisce without trying to rekindle a relationship. I told him everything—how I had gained so much weight, become depressed, and seen a psychiatrist. He was always a good listener, but what he said next surprised me.

"Melanie, don't take this the wrong way, but you're too pretty to be fat."

Was he paying me a compliment or insulting me? At 235 pounds, I knew I was the heaviest medical student in the class, male or female. I was also aware of the health consequences of being obese, and I wanted to be a good role model for Jonathan. But maybe Albert had a point.

Walking around the hospital one day, I saw a flyer for WEIGHT WATCHERS AT WORK, a weekly meeting for Stanford employees. I liked the Weight Watchers approach, which emphasized a lifestyle change rather than quick weight loss schemes, some of which I'd already tried. "This just might work!" I thought. The meetings were held at lunchtime, so I wouldn't have to worry about childcare. I was finally ready to do something about my problem. I'd been watching my weight all right—watching it go up and up and up. I would have to pay the usual fees since I wasn't technically an employee of Stanford, but the woman in charge told me I was welcome to join.

The meetings were held in a conference room in an administrative area of the hospital, tucked away from places where most of the medical students congregated for lunch, so I could join the program with a degree of privacy. In fact, I was actually glad to get away from the usual medical student lunchtime gossip and be around other people who shared the common goal of losing weight.

I was the heaviest member of the group, and eighty pounds from being at the highest weight at which I could be considered healthy. I had a long way to go, but I had to begin somewhere.

* * *

21

I finally made it through the pre-clinical years after endless hours of studying. Even though I had conquered the first two years of medical training, the clinical years would represent another world, a radical shift in emphasis calling for me to actually be responsible for the care of live patients. It was not going to be an easy apprenticeship because there are several "players" in the field hierarchy on the wards. There would be interns, or first-year residents, as well as more experienced residents. Above them were the fellows, students involved in advanced training in their chosen field, and lastly were the attendings, who at the apex of the hierarchy, were physicians with years of experience.

At teaching hospitals such as Stanford, attendings usually enjoy teaching and are also involved in research, writing articles or book chapters, and giving lectures. Because they are extremely busy in these various activities, it is a given that students respect the hierarchy. The allocation of duties is as follows: medical students collect and report data to the intern; the intern takes this data, devises a possible treatment plan, writes orders, and gives his recommendations to the resident; being more experienced, the resident guides both the interns and the medical students beneath them; and finally, the attending gives approval for any particular treatment plan. It is the attending who is naturally responsible for the actions of everyone below him or her.

It is difficult being a medical student on the wards since he or she is low on the totem pole. Medical students must be literally present to assist interns and residents when asked to do so, but their chores are somewhat mundane: they read lab values, listen to the heart and lungs, and assist in any procedures when requested. At the same time, they are expected not to get in the way of nurses or get underfoot during emergencies, such as when a patient codes. When an emergency developed, I would usually be in the very back of the room, my function being no more lofty than handing a resident his rubber gloves.

Still, there were times I felt on top of the world. I was proud to wear my white coat and a stethoscope. Each new year of clinical training begins in July, and I was still easing my way into the hierarchy in September, but I had survived the grueling class work of the first two years. Not all of my friends had been so lucky.

I was also learning how to play the game, so to speak. The clinical years involve rotations through various specialties in medicine, such as internal medicine, surgery, psychiatry, ophthalmology, dermatology, oncology, OB/GYN, and others. Students can also take elective rotations, such as anesthesiology, radiology, or pathology. But there is a definite strategy involved in choosing which rotations (each lasting a month or two) to begin with in July. I knew that medical students and interns are not very knowledgeable when the first clinical year begins, so I decided to start with a rotation in clinical medicine rather than my intended specialty, which was OB/GYN. If I were incompetent and fumbling, I would not likely receive glowing letters of recommendation from the doctors on that rotation. I wanted to feel comfortable presenting the patients to the intern, resident, and attending by the time I got to obstetrics. The residents and interns would also be more experienced themselves later in the year, and that meant I would also learn more about the specialty.

The need for such a strategy, however, goes beyond wanting to simply "look good" on the wards. To be allowed into a residency program for a desired specialty, medical students must apply to various programs while in their fourth year of medical school. They submit applications, together with letters of recommendation, to the program they desire and then interview for their desired specialty. They submit a "rank list" to the National Residency Matching Program—NRMP—while the residency programs submit their own lists of preferred candidates to the NRMP. A computer at the NRMP then "matches" the medical students with various programs.

While the process is actually far more complicated than this, the germane point is that a specialty is not simply there for the asking for students who have completed medical school. There is stiff competition and jockeying for position while a student goes through the various rotations.

*　*　*

My clinical years therefore started with internal medicine. My intern was Steve, and my resident was Bobby. They went out of their way to find a good "medical student case" for me—my very *first* case. They aimed for someone with a diagnosis that would be interesting but not esoteric or overwhelming for a new clinical student.

My first patient was named Jimmy Scotts, a fifty-five-year-old man who had a history of alcoholism and liver failure. Upon entering his room for the first time, I immediately saw the most obvious symptoms of the disease: pale yellow skin indicating jaundice, and a protuberant abdomen. Such distension of the abdomen is caused by a collection of fluid called ascites, or toxins that a diseased liver can no longer metabolize. These become systemic and cause mental disorientation, which is why Mr. Scotts was usually mumbling incoherently whenever I entered his room.

Several monitors and tubes were attached to his body, and I felt uncomfortable, as if I were an intruder on what was most certainly a death scene. Steven had informed me that the prognosis for this patient was bleak, and I didn't really have enough information to help Mr. Scotts. If these were the man's final days, however, then I might have the opportunity to save someone else's life in the future by learning as much as I could about Mr. Scotts. He was unaware of my presence, so I was free to study his chart at length to ascertain his complete case history and prior courses of treatment. Despite all I had learned in my pathology classes, scanning the many medical terms and acronyms on his chart seemed like reading a foreign language. It was one in which I would become fluent, however, in a very short time.

"We need to tap him today," Steven informed me.

"Tap him?" I said.

"Yes. We have to remove the fluid from abdomen in a procedure called paracentesis."

My mind instantly filled with questions: how was this done, and more importantly, who would do it? Would the procedure be performed by Steven, Bobby, or the attending? Would I be watching, and if so, how gross was it going to be? I was only a medical student and the "yuck factor" was a consideration. How much could my stomach handle? This was going to be an intense and rapid immersion into the real practice of medicine, but I knew that, over time, I would get used to the distinct smells and sights of dying patients. I had grown accustomed to the stench and filth caused by Darryl when we lived in Stead, so I suppose that my training for such scenes had begun earlier than I had realized. Indeed, if Darryl kept drinking the way he had during the years I'd known him, he would become another Jimmy Scotts.

A few hours later, I watched Bobby and Steve perform the tap. Fortunately, both the patient and I survived the procedure, and I was in awe of Bobby's confidence. Would I ever be as calm and assured as he was? Of course I would, but I realized that I would need to work my way through many more patients before I acquired the poise of Bobby.

As he was wrapping up, Steven said, "Read up on hepatic encephalopathy tonight."

It was already 7 p.m., and I had to be back at the hospital the next morning at 6:30. How was I supposed to read up on hepatic encephalopathy, learn the appropriate medical acronyms and other abbreviations, read up on "taps," spend time with Jonathan, and attend Weight Watchers? It was like trying to do a European tour of ten countries in two days.

I was simultaneously exhilarated and exhausted. For the time being, I would have to hope that the pounds I'd lost would stay off as I kicked into high gear to see patients on the wards, keep up with Jonathan, and do the necessary research into various procedures and diseases. It was overwhelming, but I was learning a great deal and maybe I would burn the fat by staying in perpetual motion.

* * *

I wanted Mark to be as happy as possible while staying with us. I wished I knew more about his business so I could contribute something substantive to our conversations. I attempted to be easygoing and laid-back so he would continue to be Jon's "manny," but I also wanted him to see that I was an easy person to be in a relationship with—if only he were interested! Ironically, he even told me I should not be hesitant in speaking up regarding any concerns I might have. He'd lost Jonathan at a baseball game—Jon went to a police officer and everything turned out fine—but I knew that Mark was trustworthy. My real "concerns" were about my crush on him, which I knew would eventually pass, but in the meantime I didn't want to make Mark uncomfortable. I therefore didn't speak up, putting Jon's needs first.

My depression was easing up, and I was sleeping better. I felt as if a great weight had been lifted from my shoulders—the same feeling as losing *real* weight and knowing that a goal has been accomplished.

I felt very relaxed with the young psychiatry resident, Dr. Teaford, that I'd been referred to. He was not somebody I originally thought I could relate to—he had red hair, freckles, and a pale complexion, a sharp contrast to my own appearance—but I had decided to give therapy a real chance. From the beginning, he was accepting of the things I had to say. He didn't just recite a lot of maxims, such as "you should exercise or eat right." Instead, he challenged me to acknowledge what I thought and believed. I shared with him my feelings about Darryl, Jonathan, my mother, and my sister. And even though I didn't think he'd understand, I also shared with him my feelings about being a minority student and single mom in medical school. It was almost as if I were testing him. I shared my inner-most thoughts with my journal and with God, but would a stranger, even though he was a professional, be able to understand the practical side of my worries and concerns. Was his background too far removed from my own experiences?

Dr. Teaford, as it turned out, really heard me. He understood where I was coming from. There was no right or wrong in his assessments, just "It's okay to be the way you are."

Nevertheless, I was embarrassed to tell him about Mark, but I trusted him, so I worked up my nerve and literally forced the words out of my mouth.

"Mark, my babysitter, boarder—whatever you want to call him—helps me with Jonathan, and he's so nice and caring. He likes sports, is responsible, is starting his own company, and is great with Jonathan. He's positive and encourages me to go out more. And he's ambitious."

I continued, smiling with sadness as I enumerated his qualities.

"And . . ." I paused. "I have some feelings for him." I paused a second time. "But I can't have these feelings because the arrangement is good for my son. I really want to make these feelings stop. I can't have them while he's living with us."

I told Dr. Teaford how I was trying to learn more about his business and also be a good cook. I confided that I was even a tad bit jealous at times, wondering who Mark was talking to on the phone. Sometimes, I told him, I would feel giddy just brushing past him in the hallway.

My therapist was totally sympathetic in his responses as he guided me through my feelings with a series of comments and questions.

"It's no surprise you have these feelings for him, Melanie," Dr. Teaford said. "And it's perfectly okay to have those feelings. Looking at your past, it's understandable why you would want to have someone like that in your life."

"But I can't have these feelings unless they are reciprocated," I countered. "Maybe he really likes me but can't make a move because of the situation, you know? Maybe it's up to me to let him know."

I knew I was being unrealistic even as I spoke the words, but I wanted to hear how Dr. Teaford would respond. Was there even a faint glimmer of hope?

He didn't feed my unrealistic expectations, however.

"Imagine Jonathan having a crush on his twenty-five-year-old preschool teacher," he said, pausing afterward to let the scenario fully sink into my mind. "Would you tell him he's a bad person for having a crush on her?"

"No, I wouldn't."

"Would you tell him ways to get his teacher to like him?"

"No, because it would be unrealistic."

"Then what would you tell him, Melanie? How would you respond to his feelings?"

"I'm not sure."

"You'd be gentle with him. You would likely reinforce that he's a great person and that he'll find a suitable partner in the future."

My therapist's words were hard to hear, but I appreciated his perspective and honesty. I was finally able to think about the situation in an entirely new way. That didn't stop me, however, from praying that Mark would find a girlfriend soon so he would be officially "off limits."

* * *

Mark visited his family on the east coast for the holidays, which afforded me the opportunity, as Dr. Teaford put it, to "wean myself" off him. Unfortunately, Mark's trip coincided with finals. I wasn't sure what to do since Jonathan had two birthday parties to attend in just one weekend. I bought gifts, wrapped them, and had Jon sign the cards. I wanted to just drop Jonathan off at the parties and be notified of when it was time to pick him up since the "study cloud" was hanging over my head, but the parents put in a great deal of preparation and time for the parties, and I didn't want Jonathan to miss out on any of the activities.

I called Mom and told her about the situation. I'd been in medical school long enough to know that we'd gotten beyond the "I should have stayed in Reno" speech. She saw that I was succeeding as a single mother in medical school. Mom asked when I'd be visiting her next, and I related my quandary over finals and told he that I was also involved with a research project on cervical cancer screening. I would therefore be working during the winter break.

"How about sending Jonathan out here for the break?" she suggested.

I couldn't just drive to Reno for four hours and then return, nor did I think that my Escort would necessarily make it through the snow without mechanical trauma. Besides, every spare hour had to be devoted to my finals and research.

"I don't think I can make it, Mom."

I had already promised myself that I would never resort to traveling by Greyhound bus again if at all possible. In fact, it would take even longer to reach Reno by bus because of the Greyhound's frequent stops.

"Have him fly," Mom said with no hesitation. "Kids do it all the time."

Was this my mother talking? I looked down at Jon, who returned the gaze, curious about the strange conversation.

"Jonathan on a plane by himself?"

"The flight attendants will help. Call the airlines and look into it. I'd like to see my grandson before he graduates from high school."

I could only laugh. I wanted to tell Mom that airplanes, buses, and interstates made transportation possible both ways. She was perfectly free to come visit us. I knew that this was not my mother's style, however. If anything, I was grateful that she was offering to help out.

Southwest Airlines told me that Jonathan, at five, could fly by himself as an unaccompanied minor. Since it was a nonstop flight, I could bring him to the gate, and my mother would be waiting at the other end to greet him as soon as he stepped off the plane. It was a good plan that covered all the bases, so I charged the ticket on my credit card. A few days later, Jonathan and I headed to the San Jose Airport for his first solo flight. He wore his green striped sweater since that was his "favoritest" thing to wear, as were a pair of bright blue rain boots Mark had given him for Christmas. Jon's Scooby Doo pack was filled with animal crackers, crayons, and stickers to keep him occupied on the short flight.

"Bye, Jon-Jon," I said at the gate, holding back tears as I gave him a final hug and a kiss on the cheek.

"Bye, Mommy," Jonathan said, waving.

The flight attendant assured me things would be just fine.

"Nana will be waiting for you at the airport," I said, trying to be enthusiastic. "She can't wait to see you."

He smiled, and I was surprised when the male flight attendant held out his hand and Jonathan grasped it as they walked down the rampway to the plane. I stood in place in case he looked back, which he did. He seemed excited about his adventure, regarding it as a forty-minute Disneyland ride.

I watched the plane pull away from the gate. I prayed for a safe flight, grateful that my mother was stepping up to help me again. I had proved to her and myself that I was capable of following my dreams.

* * *

As it turned out, Mark realized that his start-up company was not going to be the next Google and that he would have to find regular employment. He also found a girlfriend, which enabled me to move past my crush on him with finality.

But with Mark moving out to be with his girlfriend, I needed another manny. After a few rough starts, I hired Ian, who was studying for his PhD in chemistry. Ian was the opposite of Mark in that he was less of a jock and more domestic. He was a vegetarian and exposed Jonathan and me to different cuisines that we'd never tried before. He also understood that I had to put in long hours at the hospital and didn't mind picking up Jonathan from school. He and his girlfriend Anna, who visited occasionally and was also very nice, helped Jonathan out with creative projects for school. In general, they enjoyed hanging out with Jonathan, and I was happy that he was getting exposure to some really great people.

* * *

Jonathan started kindergarten in the fall of 1999. On his first day, we rode our bikes together to the Escondido Elementary School. He looked happy on his bicycle, Scooby Doo pack on his back. Many parents were there for this milestone in their children's lives, and although some of the children were naturally crying, Jonathan was able to say goodbye to me just fine.

A few weeks into school, Jonathan's teacher called to say that she was concerned that he didn't know his numbers and colors as well as he should by age five. I told her about Jon's speech delay and his attendance at the Special Children's Clinic in Reno, asking her what kind of resources were presently available to him. Fortunately, the school had a team approach, and I met with the school's principal, psychologist, counselor, and teacher, bringing all of his previous records to the meetings. An IEP, or individualized educational plan, was put in place, and things worked out great.

Jonathan was such a wonderful kid. I got down on the floor with him one day and hugged him as we rolled around and played. I wanted to do everything possible to be his advocate, and I wanted him to be able to look back at his childhood and say, "You did a great job, Mom!"

Things were difficult at times, but I'd come a long way. I knew I was going to make it through medical school, and Jonathan seemed off to a good start. I'd made the right decision in keeping him. And I'd shown everyone, my mother most of all, that I was capable of doing almost anything when I set my mind to it. I'd lost weight, conquered depression, and been admitted to medical school. Not bad for a young woman who was once a single mother in high school in Jackson. I'd been abused, judged, and labeled.

But I was now well on my way to being Dr. Watkins. That was the label that counted the most next to "good mom."

* * *

22

Medical school was all-consuming, and I myself was consuming a lot of food as well. With my weight officially on the back burner, I had gained back fifty pounds since my final pre-clinical year. I now weighed 230 pounds and was keenly aware of how an overweight medical student might be perceived by patients and peers alike, but balancing Jonathan's care and my clinical training didn't leave time for much else, so I regarded my weight issue as less of a priority. There was simply no time for eating right, exercise, or even religion—and I prayed that God, who I believed was paving my way, would understand. Sundays were spent studying or on the wards. Pastor Harrison encouraged the congregation to make house calls to the "church's medical student." Church members would stop by if a local store was running a "Buy one, get one free" sale, so I was often the recipient of the free extra product, and the care packages meant a lot to me.

* * *

Ian and I communicated via a simple paging system. 911 naturally meant "emergency. 411 meant one of us had information for the other. I received a 411 message one day and learned that Jonathan had lost a tooth in a bowl of corn. I laughed at the thought of Ian fishing through the corn in order to find the tooth, but I was sad that I had missed yet another milestone in Jonathan's growth. It was becoming common to hear of these events secondhand from Ian.

"Tell Jonathan 'congratulations'!" I told Ian.

It was the first tooth Jonathan lost, and when I got home and saw that he was fast asleep, I slid into the bed we shared and slipped a dollar under his pillow. I was mother, medical student, and tooth fairy, and these roles were about the only ones I could juggle. I craved a boyfriend, but I didn't have the time to be anyone's girlfriend, plus I figured that my weight was keeping most people at bay anyway.

* * *

I was literally learning how to be a doctor during my clinical years. Physicians are busy, confident, and move through hospitals quickly, often using the stairs to stay in shape or avoid long waits for an elevator. I was moving in fast motion as well as I tried to keep pace with my interns, residents, and attendings, but there was one time when I was reminded by God of the reason I had pursued my goals with so much fervor to begin with. I was walking briskly on my way to a medicine ward when a Philipino woman sitting on a bench called after me, saying, "I wish I could walk as fast as you." I looked back, paused, and then retraced my steps and sat next to her, chatting about why she was in the hospital.

She placed her hand on my arm and we spent a few minutes talking about her fears and anxiety over her daughter's surgery. It was a therapeutic moment for both of us. I was wrapping up my rotation in internal medicine, and I needed the reminder that I was going into medicine not only to learn sterile, "clinical" procedures, but to be a balm in people's time of need. It was to give time and understanding to patients and their families. After my brief talk with the woman, I felt better about what I was doing and realized that the stress was worth it. One day I'd be able to have more moments like this one, and that would be the biggest payoff of all.

* * *

A few weeks later, I successfully finished internal medicine, and I'd discovered that one of the most frustrating aspects of medicine in general was that there was so much to learn. In my next rotation, however, which would be OB/GYN, I would be learning the skills to bring new lives into the world, skills that would be far more rewarding than watching paracen-tisis. I was thrilled at the prospect of doing "real medicine."

While rotating through OB/GYN, all medical students have the objective of performing as many deliveries as possible. Even for those not intending to specialize in obstetrics, it is probably the only time in their lives when they will have the opportunity to deliver babies. This was doubly important to me since this was my intended specialty. Because of the match system of residency, I also knew it was important that I perform well and obtain as much experience as possible on the obstetrics ward. If I did, my letters of recommendation would be that much better.

My strategy was to do my rotation at the county hospital, Santa Clara Valley Medical Center, so as to get in more deliveries since there is a great deal of competition among interns and residents at the university hospital to do as many deliveries as possible. There was also less patient volume at the county facility, and cases were less specialized, whereas at the university hospital many cases tended to be specialized "medical student" deliveries involving various kinds of complications that required advanced training. Additionally, many physicians at Stanford also had private practices and wanted medical students as far away as possible from their patients. At Santa Clara, the staff was more accommodating to medical students, while mothers, many of whom had delivered before, simply wanted to give birth and return home as quickly as possible. Their "equipment" had already been stretched, and giving birth was usually easier for them. I was eager to start this rotation, therefore, because I was confident and knew that this would be an opportunity to shine. And on top of everything else, I had given birth myself, which was something most other medical students had not experienced.

On my first day on OB/GYN, I made sure to let as many people as possible know that this was my chosen specialty. I didn't get any deliveries the first week since it was necessary to observe a few before I was allowed to do the honors myself. That was perfectly fine with me, holding women's hands for hours while cheering them on and reminding them to push and breath.

I studied Friedman's Labor Curve, a very old but useful text on the average times a woman could be expected to remain in the various stages of labor. I therefore memorized these stages, knowing I'd be ready when the time came.

The intern on the ward was Christina, who also had to get in a large number of deliveries. She said she hadn't gotten as many as she wanted while in medical school and informed me that she would do most of the delivering. This didn't seem fair since she should have been able to empathize with my need to obtain the same experience. She'd been standing in my shoes while in medical school, and surely she could find a way to see that I, too, would be able to get a decent number of deliveries.

Nevertheless, she allowed me to deliver the placenta on many occasions, which is no simple task. A placental avulsion can occur if the placenta is pulled too hard before it has completely separated from the wall of the uterus, often causing the umbilical cord to break. When this happens, it is necessary to reach inside the uterus and physically manipulate the remaining placenta, which can precipitate heavy bleeding in the mother. I successfully delivered many placentas, but no babies.

I was frustrated. I didn't want to "tattle" on the intern, but I needed the experience as much as she did. As luck would have it, our attending was a young woman who'd graduated from Brigham, a Harvard-affiliated school, just a few years earlier. Dr. Sheila Campbell preferred us to call her by her first name, which was almost unheard of in the hierarchy, but I couldn't bring myself to do it. Even though she was young and laid-back, it seemed disrespectful. I did tell her, however, that I truly wanted to go into OB/GYN even though it was not a popular specialty because of the extended "on call" hours, plus the medical-legal concerns were considerable. Obstetricians pay some of the highest premiums for malpractice insurance of all the specialties. Dr. Campbell was pleased to hear that I wanted to go into her specialty. A great many students try to score points with an attending by claiming that each rotation will be their specialty, although most attendings see right through such claims. Perhaps because of my personal history as a single mother, Dr. Campbell saw my sincerity.

"I've delivered enough placentas, Dr. Campbell," I said, "but I need a delivery. I stay up all night when I'm on call, but it just isn't happening." I withheld my knowledge that it wasn't happening because of Christina.

"Melanie, when are you on call next?"

"Um, tomorrow night."

"Let's switch your call to a night when I'm on, too," Dr. Campbell suggested. "It will be just you and me, and we'll make sure you get your deliveries."

"Thank you!" I said. I wanted to hug her, but I knew it was inappropriate.

As I walked away, I felt a rush of fear and angst. What if I couldn't deliver a baby? What if it slipped from my arms (which often happened in delivery rooms)? What if I pulled the wrong way on the baby's head? What if I encountered a shoulder dystocia, which is when the baby gets stuck in the birth canal, or a delivery in which the cord was wrapped around the baby's neck? Dr. Campbell would be looking over my shoulder, of course, but I thought of every possible emergency that I had read about in my coursework.

The night I was on call with Dr. Campbell, the labor board, a wall-mounted board that kept track of women in labor on the ward, was almost full. This was indeed the perfect night to be on call.

The first delivery involved a Hispanic woman. This would be her third baby, so her "pipes were prepped," which meant that the delivery would most likely be quick and uncomplicated. I spoke to her in the "medical Spanish" I had learned thus far.

"Empuje! Empuje!" *Push. Push.* I smiled as I looked between her legs. A smile on such occasions was the universal language of "Good job! You're doing well!"

Her Hispanic husband was by her side, and as I looked at him, I had the feeling that was so common when I saw couples going through the miraculous process of delivery together. It was a bittersweet moment, with sadness for not having this kind of experience myself while delivering Jonathan mixed with the hope that I might find a wonderful man and still have the chance to share such a moment in the future. If the latter didn't happen, then I would continue to share in the happiness of others, cheating, as it were, while I shared vicariously in the joy of this important moment of their lives.

Dr. Campbell told me to gown and glove up. We placed a plastic bag underneath the mother's bottom while the nurse helped us get ready. It was show time.

The baby was crowning, which meant I could see the top of its head starting to emerge. Dr. Campbell whispered in my ear, gently directing me as the birth proceeded. I was really doing this, and I was so happy that I wanted to cry! The baby came out in one final push. I cradled it in my arms like a football as Dr. Campbell helped me cut the cord.

"Tiene hijo!" I exclaimed. "You have a boy!"

We handed the baby to his mother, and the father leaned over and kissed his child and his wife. I was completely in awe.

"One more step, Melanie," Dr. Campbell said, reminding me of something that should have become second nature to me.

There was the placenta to deliver.

I massaged the abdomen, which helps the placenta to contract, and it was delivered quickly. I then cleaned the mother and looked carefully at her perineum, the area beneath the vagina. I was very proud of myself since there were no tears. I finished up and washed my hands before approaching the father, who spoke more English than his wife.

"Congratulations!" I said. "You have a beautiful baby."

He was very talkative. "Do you have any children?" he asked.

"Yes, a son."

He probed further.

"And do you have a husband as well?"

The question seemed a bit intrusive, but I responded since he seemed sweet and responsive. No insult was intended.

"No, I don't."

He relayed our conversation to his wife.

"Do you have a friend?" she asked in broken English.

Culturally, it seemed very important to them that I not be "soltera," or alone. They meant well.

Dr. Campbell's pager rescued me from the awkward situation.

"Come on," she said. "We have to go."

I smiled and waved as we walked away.

There was another delivery down the hallway. And then another . . . and another. By the time the night was over, I had delivered ten babies, each one special and unique. I was exhilarated but tired.

I was glad I'd spoken to Dr. Campbell. My assertiveness had paid off.

* * *

Almost everything on the OB/GYN ward had been feminine: nurses, patients, interns, residents, and attendings. The opposite would be true for my next rotation, which was surgery at the Veterans Affairs Center. The patients and surgeons were predominantly male. Even my female attending, Dr. Julie Shaw, behaved in a noticeably masculine manner. I'd heard that she didn't like female students very much—or perhaps herself, for that matter. She was a classic case of someone very authoritative using her seniority to cover insecurity. One could look at her and tell that she'd paid her dues. She was one of the boys in every way, a no frills woman who wore no lipstick and always kept her hair pinned on top of her head. I'd heard many tales of her rough demeanor and was very intimidated in her presence. She didn't seem to like me from the very beginning, and I found myself fumbling around her—doubting myself, forgetting my words, and generally spacing out.

Her mantra in any situation was, "Melanie, this is surgery!"— a reminder that I was not performing up to her expectations. My resident, Billy Thomas, had his own problems. He was arrogant, cocky, and attractive (and he knew it), a standard Stanford resident brimming with confidence.

"Sometimes wrong, never in doubt!" he would assert.

"Yes," I would nod as I ran after him down the hallways at 6 a.m., stethoscope in hand and my surgery pocketbooks in my lab coat.

I didn't want to expose my naiveté, so I studied every one of these small manuals that I could find. One can usually tell how far advanced a medical student is by the number of books weighting down his or her pockets. At the time, I carried such pocketbooks as *Surgery: On Call* and *Surgical Recall*, and if there had been such a volume, I would have also carried *Surgery for Dummies*. I read up on every case lest I get pimped by Billy Thomas. In medicine, "pimped" is a term meaning "Put In My Place." Medical students get pimped when asked picayunish questions on the spot, ones they can't answer. There is little warning for these ambushes, and it is even worse when it happens in front of colleagues, especially on rounds. When the medical student doesn't know something, then the intern is expected to come up with the answer. If the intern gets pimped, then the resident is expected to have the answer. As always in the hierarchy, there is a chain of command that is rigidly followed—and no one ever wants to get pimped.

In surgery, I felt completely helpless. I was "the human retractor" keeping blood out of the way so that Dr. Shaw and Billy could see the surgical field.

"Melanie, this is surgery!" Dr. Shaw would emphasize, as if I needed to be reminded. "We need to be able to see the structures."

If I didn't know the four Fs for who was likely to develop gallstone— mnemonics for "fat, fifties, female, and flatulent"—it was "Melanie, this is surgery!"

When Dr. Shaw and I saw patients for consultations or pre-surgical appointments, I dreaded working with her. She had no bedside manner, being curt and to the point with all patients regardless of their illnesses. She usually looked at the chart more than at the actual patient. Her questions were frequently single words delivered in staccato fashion.

"Pain? Where? Bleeding? Quantity?"

I felt quite bad for the patients as well as myself. I was trapped with an attending who was the antithesis of the kind of doctor I wanted to be, a doctor who would have thought my rationale for being a physician was naïve in the extreme.

"Melanie," she said, "go see Mr. Burroughs."

I hated the way she spoke my name. The syllables came out as if she were annoyed by having to muster the breath just to say them. When she said, "Melanie," she exhibited profound disappointment and low expectations.

She handed me the patient's chart, and I sat down and examined it for fifteen minutes, wishing to be thorough. There were many patients, however, and the clinic was backing up.

"Melanie, get out there and see that patient. This is surgery! It's not like the Ku Klux Klan is in the waiting room."

I was taken aback. Had I heard correctly? Was Dr. Shaw racist as well as insensitive? I decided that underneath all of her meanness and grandiosity, she had to know that her remark was way out of line. She would surely take back her comment and apologize.

I swallowed hard and took the chart. As I had done on so many occasions, I stared up at the ceiling in order to keep my tears in check, as if looking to God to give me strength. I made my way to the waiting room, trying to focus on Mr. Burroughs abdominal pain, but Dr. Shaw's comment continued to distract me.

When I returned to Dr. Shaw to present the case, I realized that I'd omitted the abdominal exam—and it was too late to go back. There were too many patients waiting to be seen. The attending's next remarks were quite predictable. The screech returned with all of its unmelodic connotations.

"Melanie, this is surgery! Why didn't you examine his abdomen?"

"Well, Dr. Shaw, he was in a lot of pain, and I knew that you would be examining him, too, so I didn't want to put him through the extra discomfort."

I wanted to cry, so I looked at the wall to my right. When I turned back, Dr. Shaw glared at me incredulously.

"How could you forget to do a simple abdominal exam?"

The answer was that I was still in shock from her insensitive remark, but this wasn't something I could tell her. If I were honest, I'd risk a very bad letter of recommendation that, in turn, could radically affect the residency program to which I'd be matched.

But maybe I was making too much of the incident. Maybe she was just clueless about social interactions. Perhaps I was being oversensitive.

I called Karen to get some perspective. Karen had done her surgery rotation at the county hospital. She wanted to be a urologist and was capable of "playing tough" with the boys, even those in the male-dominated field of surgery. I would also have called Dr. Teaford, but he was wrapping up his residency and would soon be practicing as an attending in another state. Karen was therefore the only person who might be able to understand the delicate situation I was in.

Karen's opinion was unequivocal. "You need to tell the dean," she stated.

"The dean of the medical school? No, that's going too far." I suddenly wanted to put the incident behind me. Following Karen's advice might stir up a hornet's nest and ruin my entire career.

"If you don't tell him," Karen said, "I will. Attendings can't go around saying things like that. This is Stanford Medical School, and it's 2002!"

"But I'm still on surgery," I said. "You can't tell the dean. I've got to get through the rotation!"

I imagined the dean talking to the chair of surgery, who would reprimand Dr. Shaw. In turn, Dr. Shaw would retaliate by giving me low marks.

"But what about the students who are going to have her next month?" asked Karen. "She needs to know as soon as possible that she was out of line."

I began to regret telling Karen. I had opened the proverbial can of worms.

"Karen, I'll never speak to you again if you tell the dean. Never."

"That's your choice, Melanie."

Karen hung up abruptly.

I had a case with Dr. Shaw the following morning. As I scrubbed in, the lights in the adjacent operating room seemed especially bright, and the beeping of the monitors seemed abnormally loud. The right side of my head began to throb. The migraines had returned.

* * *

I decided to speak with Dr. Jackson, the only African American woman in the surgery department. I wished I had drawn her as my attending, as did many minority students, but Dr. Jackson was a newer faculty member, and most of us drew Dr. Shaw, who had far more seniority.

Dr. Jackson knew that Dr. Shaw was difficult to work with, but she encouraged me to hang in there. She reiterated that being a person of color in a predominately white field was difficult. She explained that it was necessary to practice restraint and hold back one's words from time to time in order to maintain a professional posture. She wasn't giving me specific advice on the situation, but rather validation and acknowledgement of the challenges I faced as a woman of color. She clearly understood my feelings. I got the distinct impression, however, that was telling me not to make waves—and that she wouldn't either in light of the fact that she'd only been at Stanford for a short time. Her mindset was that we both, as African American women, had to be willing to put up with occasional indignities in order to practice medicine. My quandary therefore remained, and I wondered what Karen was going to do.

I found out soon enough. Karen reported Dr. Shaw to the dean of the medical school, who relayed the incident to the chairman of surgery, as well as the surgery clerkship director (who was in charge of rotation assignments). I was extremely angry since I'd told Karen about the encounter in the strictest confidence. Why couldn't she have waited until the letters of recommendation were written?

I was summoned to speak to the dean of minority affairs and the clerkship director. They asked me what happened, and I found it difficult to look at them let alone speak. I related the incident hesitantly, but meanwhile I still had to work with Dr. Shaw on the wards.

The issue escalated into one of racism, with university lawyers becoming involved. I felt vulnerable and trapped. I wanted the dean and the chair of surgery to know that I wasn't as angry as Karen, although I was nevertheless ambivalent. I wanted people to know that I wasn't the one who'd brought Dr. Shaw's remark to light, but by the same token, I didn't want to trivialize the situation and have people believe that I didn't think it shouldn't be dealt with.

I wasn't comfortable telling Billy what had happened. For all of his bravado, he was trying to help me with my confidence and was spending valuable time teaching me. While applying steri-strips to a groggy patient's skin after removing his surgical staples, he whispered, "Melanie, you know your stuff and present well. You just need to work on your confidence."

I couldn't imagine being as confident as Billy. I would like to have confided in Billy, telling him of my dilemma with our attending, but I didn't want to taint my working relationship with him. I felt that he, too, realized how overbearing she was, and yet he never said anything disrespectful about her. I felt I should do the same and follow his lead since surgery was no place for whining. I was in the hospital one hundred hours a week, and there was no room for the touchy-feely stuff. As Dr. Shaw frequently said, "This is surgery!" It wasn't the venue for bruised egos.

* * *

I was taking Elavil to help with the daily migraines, but the med was making me so sleepy that I wasn't always able to "pre-round," or see patients before formal morning rounds because I sometimes overslept. I could barely stay awake during Grand Rounds (when someone especially important in his or her filed conducted rounds). Not wanting anyone to see me snoozing, I walked out, followed by Rachel, an eloquent and confident classmate. She saw how down I looked and was very concerned. She believed I needed to tell Dr. Shaw and Billy why I had to excuse myself, but this was unheard of. I didn't want to be viewed as a slacker. The truth was that I was slipping back into clinical depression. I was burnt out and didn't always have the time to refill my Prozac prescription. The doses were therefore skipped. I found myself jealous of those students who were carefree and had time to shoot the breeze.

But my other dilemma had not evaporated either. The following day, I met with a university representative about Dr. Shaw. I found out that I would no longer be working directly beneath her for the last three weeks of my rotation, nor would she be allowed to evaluate my performance in a letter of recommendation. I began to think that something good was going to come of this very messy situation after all. I was told that Dr. Shaw would be disciplined, although I was not, as a medical student, privy to the details of what such discipline might entail. In addition, Dr. Jackson felt motivated to become more involved in the issue. She said that I'd actually inspired her and said that she would help me organize a seminar for medical students on how to deal with issues of racism involving patients and staff.

I still wasn't talking with Karen and needed more time to process my feelings of betrayal. I had learned a few valuable life lessons from the whole debacle, but it had been very stressful, causing the migraines to continue.

I was still confident that God was directing my future. I'd learned, as the saying goes, that I didn't know what the future holds, but I knew *who* held my future.

* * *

23

The next rotation was anesthesiology. I'd sit next to the resident during surgery and watch as he jotted notes on a piece of paper every few minutes or so. At times, he'd make slight adjustments to the anesthetic agents he was administering or the machines used to monitor a patient's vital signs. I watched him for hours and hours, case after case. Once, seeing the boredom on my face, he answered the question in my mind: "Why would anyone choose this specialty?"

"Anesthesiology is not a spectator sport," he said.

Oh, I thought. Would this be more enjoyable if *I* were the one jotting down vital signs while the patient was unconscious?

The monitors were beeping, and I could barely make out what the surgeons were saying to each other on the other side of the surgical drape. The anesthesiologist's side was not nearly as exciting as the surgeons' side, where an actual procedure was being performed, but in many ways, this rotation felt like the break I needed. I'd had enough excitement on my surgery rotation.

"You'd probably like it more as an attending," he told me. "And, you know, it is on the road to happiness."

"What's the road to happiness?"

"Radiology, ophthamology, anesthesiology, and dermatology. All four are specialties in which the pay is great, and you get on the road home before dark. Because of that, they are some of the most competitive specialties."

He was indeed proud to have earned a position in the driver's seat on the R.O.A.D. to happiness, as it is known in medicine. He applauded himself for choosing a field like anesthesiology, one that made *me* want to go to sleep instead of putting *others* to sleep. I then wondered if, as an OB/GYN, would I be working five to nine instead of nine to five?

It was February 2002, and Jonathan had been practicing for weeks for his class Valentine's Tea. All of the mommies (and, this being Palo Alto, some nannies as well) were invited to the second graders' tribute to the special women in their lives. I was on a case that I was hoping would be done by 9:30 a.m., so I'd have time to break away for the Valentine's Tea. Jonathan never asked me for much—he knew the phrase "Mommy's busy" oh too well—but I could tell he really wanted me to be there. The case was taking longer than expected, and I frantically looked at the time on my pager: 9:10, 9:16, 9:35. It was important for me to be seen as a medical student, but I didn't necessarily want all the attendings and residents to know I was a single mother. I didn't want them to think I would be difficult or ask for special treatment, such as a day off because my child was home sick or asking to leave early. I hadn't let them know about the Valentine's Tea, and I was just hoping to ride my bike to the other side of campus to attend Jonathan's performance and get back in time for the next case. I thought I had it timed just right, but there were complications. As a medical student, you want to be around for complications. The doctor is needed when things go wrong, and medical students learn more when that happens.

The patient, who was having an appendectomy, had a difficult time coming out of the anesthesia. It was now 9:42 a.m. This was not the time to tell my resident—and the attending, who had been summoned as the patient was being awakened—that I had promised to attend my son's performance.

9:55 a.m. I came to the realization that I'd be late or might not make it at all.

"Dammit, wake up!" I said under my breath.

I was mad at a patient I didn't even know. I was mad at Jonathan's teacher for scheduling the performance at an awkward time that was not good for working moms or moms in school. I was mad at myself for being mad, which was my usual pattern.

10:14. The patient finally woke up, and all was fine. I excused myself, saying I was going to the bathroom. The next case would be at 11:30, and I'd have to be back by 11 a.m. to prep. Wearing my blue Stanford Medical Center scrubs, I hopped on my bike and pedaled as fast as a woman weighing 235 pounds could. Maybe I'd catch some of the performance.

I arrived dripping in sweat, and I didn't take the time to wipe down in the bathroom. In the classroom, the mothers, nannies, and teachers were clapping. It was 10:30 a.m. I'd missed the performance. Tears mixed with my perspiration, and I clapped briefly and halfheartedly while waving to Jonathan and to his teacher. I wiped away my tears and sweat, and Jonathan left his classmates to came over.

"Mommy! You're here!"

The other mommies, who had already finished enjoying their tea and cookies, were beginning to depart.

Jonathan's teacher announced to the class, "Let's have a repeat of the performance. An encore. We know Jonathan's mommy isn't able to make it to the classroom much, so let's do it again!"

Her words were superficially sweet but their tone had the hint of an edge. No, I wasn't able to make it there much. I brushed that off and sat in a too-tiny chair for the performance—for an audience of one.

I smiled at each of the students. Jonathan was in the front row and sang his heart out, louder than all the others. His teacher, Ms. Thomas, took a photo of Jonathan and me afterwards. Jonathan was beaming. I kissed him on the cheek and told him his performance was "Fan-tas-tic!" I clapped with every syllable and thanked Ms. Thomas. I was happy to have seen the performance that Jonathan had worked so hard on, but I knew I had to go. I biked back to the medical center. The next patient was being wheeled to the operating room as I arrived.

* * *

Something had to be done about the migraines, which were still very persistent in my post-surgery rotation. Rachel continued to encourage me to take care of myself. She didn't have children, she wasn't a minority, and she wasn't young, but something from her life experiences made her concerned for me and connected to me. She was trying to look out for my best interests even if I couldn't look out for them myself.

"You should see Dr. Blakely. We're working on a research project together. I'm sure she'd squeeze you into clinic. You really need to get some help with this, Melanie. My gosh, you've been having migraines, since..."

"Since I was thirteen," I said, finishing her sentence.

"Well, if anyone can figure out a way to help you, Dr. Blakely can."

Dr. Blakely was an esteemed neurologist, well known on the campus. She was the "triple threat" of academic neurology: She conducted research and had published in leading academic journals; she saw patients in the neurology clinic; and she taught medical students on the neurology rotation.

"But she's so busy," I countered. "I don't know."

"I'll ask her if she can see you. I know she will."

Rachel was there for me, looking out for my best interests. She leaned in and hugged me, and for a moment, I felt that she was not just a good friend, but a loving mother and protective sister, all in one.

* * *

Neurology was not a required rotation for me as a student going into obstetrics and gynecology. I would never be working directly with Dr. Blakely on the wards in the hospital, but when I saw her, I started to wish I could. The nurse placed me in a waiting room. Wearing a long white coat, Dr. Blakely, a blond woman with short hair and thin-rimmed glasses, came in a few minutes later. She had a better bedside manner than I had anticipated.

She looked down at my chart. "Let's see, Melanie Watkins." She sat on the rolling medical chair and came in close as I sat on the examining table. "So, Dr. Watkins, what seems to be the problem?" She smiled, acknowledging that I was the student Rachel had referred and giving me a title that I was three months shy of earning. I liked her instantly.

"Migraines." I sighed as I said the word, as if this was my last stop, my last chance to get some help with this recurring problem. What if migraines prevented me from being able to practice medicine?

"Migraines," she repeated.

"Yes." And instead of doing what I originally planned to do, which was to describe myself as I would a patient in the usual format—*"Twenty-three-year-old African-American woman who presents with a chief complaint of migraines. Onset. Duration. Frequency. Triggers. Remitting factors"* —I allowed myself to be a patient and began, as many patients do, with the whole story. I couldn't help it. She seemed so caring and inviting. I told her that I'd had the migraines since I was thirteen, that I had tried numerous medications, and that I worried something else might be going on. Could I have a brain tumor? I also shared a fear that was even more likely than a brain tumor: that I was scared I wouldn't be able to become an obstetrician/gynecologist and perform surgeries. What if I had a migraine as an attending? I couldn't just walk away to a dark, quiet place for an hour.

She listened to me as if she had all the time in the world, but as a medical student, I imagined she had many patients to see, as well as interns and residents waiting in the hallway, eager to get her input on their cases. But, for those fifteen minutes, I was all that she seemed to care about. She listened to all my fears and addressed my concerns.

"Can I get an MRI?" I asked.

She smiled. "A brain tumor is unlikely, but yes, I will order an MRI. I was a medical student once." She winked.

I couldn't imagine her as a medical student. Would I ever have that poise, that certainty, that confidence?

"And I'm going to give you a course of steroids. This should help. Call the clinic if you are not feeling better over the next few days."

I smiled and thanked her. It was an awkward moment. I wondered if we should shake hands as medical colleagues or just nod and say goodbye as patient and doctor. Or, as women, should I hug her? Instead, as I stood up, she placed her hand on my back and walked with me toward the door.

I took the Prednisone and began to have fewer migraines, and then they stopped altogether. I also managed to get the MRI of my head, and it was normal. The test result reassured me, plus it was a good experience, not only because I knew I didn't have brain cancer, but because I got a taste of the procedure my patients went through. I had wondered what they experienced in the MRI scanner—to be still for the entire time while layered images of their brains were being made. I now knew why patients felt claustrophobic during head imaging.

I sat down and hand-wrote a letter to Dr. Blakely, thanking her for her extra attention and care, letting her know that she was the kind of doctor I wanted to be. I placed the letter in the faculty mailbox at the university.

A few months later, while I was finishing my last rotation of medical school, Rachel called me one night. She was crying. The next words from her mouth affected me for many years to come: "Dr. Blakely committed suicide today."

Not Dr. Blakely! Was Rachel sure? Maybe Dr. Blakely had been murdered instead.

Rachel continued to sob. "She jumped off the Golden Gate Bridge." And with that, Rachel answered my question.

"Rachel, why? Why would she do that?"

I felt sadness, anger, betrayal, and disbelief. I was sad to lose someone I'd only met once. For good or bad, every attending left his or her mark on me as a young medical student. Sometimes it was only by showing me behavior I did not want to emulate. At best, as with Dr. Blakely, it was by modeling the kind of physician I wanted to be. Her death—her suicide— along with other interactions with patients and attendings, made me question my commitment to the field I'd chosen at the beginning of medical school. How could this very accomplished woman choose to end her life? What could have happened to her that was so sad and so horrible that she, an educated professional woman, would do this?

"Dr. Blakely was . . ." Rachel paused. "Well, I think she suffered from depression. She was lonely. She was in training a long time to get her M.D. and her PhD and had to play the game with the good ole boys to break the glass ceiling. I think that when she made it to professor, she must've looked back and thought 'I have no husband, I have no children, I'm fifty years old, and I just have this title—professor.' For her, that wasn't enough."

What I wanted to say, but didn't, was, "But she had us."

Dr. Blakely had medical students, and the study of medicine had a strange corollary with family. Medical students saw attendings as mothers and fathers from whom they sought approval. Selfishly, I thought, we weren't enough, and my heartfelt, handwritten thank-you card wasn't enough, either.

* * *

24

Harvard Medical School offers visiting clerkships to students of color interested in its residency programs. In the summer of 2002, I persuaded Mom to keep Jonathan so that I would be able to spend a month doing an advanced clinical rotation in Boston at one of the Harvard-affiliated hospitals. Mom had recently remarried, which was one of the best things that ever happened to her or to our relationship. She had mellowed a bit. Jonathan enjoyed his new grandfather, even saying, "Grandpa, I'm so glad I met you," which made us all laugh. I liked the fact that he now had another positive male influence.

Jonathan flew to Reno, and later in the evening, I took my flight to Boston. I had never been there before, and I looked forward to the opportunity of seeing how I would perform at another institution. I wouldn't have to worry about childcare, and although I would miss Jonathan, I was eager to focus solely on my studies and performance. Also, I would make connections in Boston and, I hoped, secure an interview.

An advanced rotation is called a sub-internship. I would be doing my sub-internship in maternal-fetal medicine, also known as high-risk obstetrics. This would involve seeing pregnant women with pre-existing medical concerns, and women with medical complications as a result of their pregnancies.

Because I would be there for a month, I moved into one of the dormitories on campus. As I walked inside, suitcase in tow, I thought back to the summer before my first year of college, when I stayed with Sarah in the dorm at the University of Nevada. There, I'd pretended that I was a student just like everyone else. I pretended that I didn't have to cope with the struggles of parenting. And here, eight years later, I was resuming that role of "just student." I was grateful to my mother for allowing me to give this my all, without any distractions.

During the first few weeks of the rotation, I was observing more than doing. The hierarchy was rigid, and I had to line up behind attendings, fellows, residents, and interns. But I learned a lot from just watching: how to support the perineum (a delicate area of tissue below the vagina) so that a woman wouldn't tear during delivery; how to tell a patient that there was a fetal demise (death); and how to obtain consent from a patient for a procedure. I was learning how to be a doctor.

I spent my downtime practicing tying my knots—one-handed ties and two-handed ties. I was happy when I had the opportunity to practice suturing. Initially, I'd sutured a folded, blue surgical towel, pretending it was a patient's incision while delicately using my needle driver to bring the ends together. I wanted to be ready if I was ever given the opportunity to suture a real patient.

That opportunity came in the third week of my rotation. Dr. Allison, one of the high-risk attendings, had a triplet delivery. I'd never seen triplets delivered, so I read up on all the possible complications during and after delivery of multiples. I was not expecting to do much. At academic institutions such as Stanford and Harvard, medical students are not very "hands on," but the experience of learning from experts in the field is unparalleled. To my surprise, Dr. Allison, a woman in her forties who was a female maternal-fetal-medicine attending at the hospital, nodded to me and placed the surgical instruments, needle driver, and forceps in my hands. She was allowing me to close part of the fascia, the subcutaneous tissue, and to finish with subcuticular stitches on the final incision, which patients often regard as the most important layer because the result is the scar that will show.

I intently focused on what I was doing, ignoring the beeping monitors and the other people in the room. I was glad I had practiced my two-handed knot-tying and that I had the opportunity to show my stuff. I may have been showing a bit of frustration, too—perhaps an "oops" here or a "shoot" there—and my attending leaned towards me and whispered, "Don't show your disappointment. Your patient and her husband are still awake." I nodded. I still had a lot to learn about being a doctor.

During my rotation, I met with the residency training director, Dr. Beecher. This was just short of an interview, and it carried the same weight and anxiety. Dr. Beecher said, "This program is not for those going into private practice." Rather, the program was intended for those entering academia—teaching and research. I wasn't quite sure if that was what I wanted, but the possibility of training at such an esteemed institution was alluring. Could I possibly make it through a four-year obstetrics and gynecology residency and a three-year maternal-fetal-medicine fellowship? The thought of seven more years of training was daunting, but so far, I'd taken things step-by-step and day-by-day. I was eight years into this, and I couldn't and wouldn't turn back.

* * *

Rotation ended. In Boston, I had managed to lose my cell phone and an earring, but hadn't lost what I wanted to lose most: weight. The stress of trying to be at the top of my game, to shine, and to be a superstar was intense and led to many trips to great East Coast delis and fast food chains. We didn't have Dunkin' Donuts on the West Coast, and it had become one of my favorite hangouts while in Boston. Before I came home, I ate what I swore was my last donut ever, and I picked up a Game Boy for Jonathan, and a gift to send my niece Sloane for her thirteenth birthday. Tonya was pregnant—expecting her second child. Time was flying by.

I flew to Reno, not only to pick up Jonathan, but to visit with my mom, my stepfather, Edward, and friends and mentors. Dr. Thornton, who continued to pay for Jonathan's childcare, invited me over, and we made cookies for Jonathan and her grandchildren. She gave me a book on meditation and signed it, "With love, affection and admiration." She was empowering and told me that I could change the world. She was such a blessing.

Sarah's life had changed dramatically. While I was in medical school in the Bay Area, Sarah had married a Laotian man. They'd struggled with infertility. She took Clomid, a medication to help her conceive, and was surprised to have triplets. When I saw her, the triplets were a year old. I thought back to our days in the dorm during the summer of 1994. Our lives were so different now. I asked about her academic goals, and she said, "Maybe five years from now, I'll go to grad school," but her voice didn't have the conviction or certainty that I was used to hearing from her. She seemed fulfilled being a "mother of multiples."

We didn't want our visit to end. We decided to call Ms. King and invite her to dinner. Sarah's husband offered to watch all the children—their three plus Jonathan. Jonathan was happy to play big brother and help out. Sarah, Ms. King, and I dined at a popular Mexican restaurant in downtown Reno. We talked about school, life, and love. It was wonderful to see Ms. King, and she was happy to see her "Hughesians." Sarah bought Jonathan one of his favorite books from the Captain Underpants series, and she nearly cried when we left, which almost made me cry.

* * *

When I returned to Palo Alto, I again faced my anxiety about the future. I was confident that I was going into obstetrics and gynecology, but where would I train? This decision was not entirely up to me; it would be part of the match. But how should I order my rank list? I had met nice attendings in Boston, one of whom had even offered to let me stay with her when I came back for formal interviews, but would I have enough support in Boston? The summer there was humid but tolerable. The winters on the East Coast could be quite harsh, and that would mean challenges with getting to work, getting Jonathan to school, and getting up earlier. And what would I do for childcare? My mind was spinning with ideas. UCSF seemed like a logical choice. UCSF and Brigham were two of the highest-rated obstetrics and gynecology training programs in the country.

I decided on a two-week gyn rotation with Dr. Grier who was a gynecologist who worked with a UCSF-affiliated hospital. He was known for his teaching, but he was also known to "pimp"—the acronym for "Put In My Place," meaning that he often reminded students of how much they didn't know. He incessantly pimped me on ovarian cysts, about which my memory was vague because I had recently focused on obstetrics, not gynecology. And the thoughts came: "I am too sensitive. I doubt myself. I need to read more. Will I ever know enough?"

At home I drowned my thoughts in a big bowl of cereal and whole milk, a pattern all too familiar to me. The fact that Jonathan was observing my unhealthy eating habits—eating out often and consuming fast food and TV dinners—compounded my guilt. Carrying around eighty extra pounds was tiring, but as much as I hated being fat, I didn't hate it enough to do anything about it. I didn't have time, and there was no end in sight. Internship would be more stressful than medical school. Residency would be more stressful than all of my previous training. Residency would mean being on call, kissing social life goodbye for ages twenty-six to twenty-nine, and using my hours away from the hospital just to hang with Jonathan, study, and sleep.

I decided I'd rejoin Weight Watchers when my rotations were less intense. The latter half of the final year of medical school would consist of lighter rotations, electives, and interviews. I wanted to lose weight for interviews and graduation in order to present myself in the best possible light. I prayed to God that I could lose the weight and be calm and confident during interviews.

* * *

25

My academic advisor suggested that I take an advanced medicine rotation. As an obstetrician/gynecologist, I would need to know how to manage non-OB/GYN concerns—diabetes, hypertension, and so on. This was especially true because more and more women were seeing their OB/GYN as their "pcp," or primary care physician. For this challenging rotation, I was expected to perform at the level of an intern, a title I would have in less than a year. As I progressed through this demanding sub-internship, I became more and more resentful of people who appeared to have a life. I was envious of others who seemed so carefree, having pastries and coffee at Starbucks, going for a morning run, socializing, and laughing.

My tenth-grade idealism of becoming a doctor faltered each morning with the buzz of the alarm at 4:30 a.m. What had made me think I could actually do this? Nothing worth having is easy, but I wondered if I really could make it through. My life consisted of nothing but school, study, sleep, and seeing Jonathan. There wasn't time for anything else. Fortunately, Stanford had a pass/fail system for both the preclinical and the clinical years, which relieved a lot of the pressure that most medical students experience. At some other medical schools, a student had the option to strive for "honors," a mark above a simple "pass." I was glad I didn't have to worry about that. My classmates and I were grateful that we were not ranked as a class; Stanford's policy decreased competitiveness among students. Still, we often joked, "What do they call the student who graduates at the bottom of her medical school class?" The answer was "doctor." I didn't feel I was at or near the bottom, but I also wondered if I ever would have been at honors level if we'd had that evaluation system at Stanford.

By this time, I had survived a second round of exams called the USMLE (United States Medical Licensing Exam), largely based on knowledge I had acquired during the clinical years of medical school (pediatrics, internal medicine, obstetrics and gynecology, surgery, and so on). Soon it would be time to apply to residency programs through the match. On the same day, usually in March of each year, the nation's medical students learn where they will spend the new few years of training. On a rank order list, the medical students rank the programs they are interested in, and the residency programs also rank the students who interest them. Then a computerized system matches students with a residency program. I needed to complete the rank order list soon. I, like many other medical students across the country, struggled with the list and the accompanying anxiety of not really knowing where I would be in July, 2003.

The first step was to get an interview with the residency programs. After all the interviews are done, the students rank the programs from their top choices on down through the NRMP (National Residency Match Program). Both medical schools and residency programs like to brag about getting their top one or two choices in "the match". Students from top schools are expected to match into their top choices of programs. Residency programs do not like the idea of going too far down the list—getting residents they weren't particularly interested in.

The scariest aspect of the match is that you don't know how the residency program director and staff feel about you, so you don't have a good idea of how to rank the programs to maximize your chances of getting the one you want. The other frightening aspect is that once you are matched, you are committed—you must attend that program. There is no changing your mind after match day.

This process was overwhelmingly anxiety-provoking for me as a single parent because it meant Jon and I could end up anywhere. We had created our support system at Stanford despite not having any family in the area, but would we be able to do that somewhere else?

I felt very lonely in making the decision by myself. Some of my classmates had spouses to assist with research on the neighborhoods of the residency programs they were considering. Spouses helped make new friends, find good schools for their children, and generally aid in the adjustment to a new area. I wished for someone to help me make this major life decision. At the same time, as frustrated I was about my single status, I was reluctant to date, even though I would have a lighter schedule after the medicine sub-internship. What if I met someone local who wanted me to stay in the Bay Area? I tried looking at the upside of being single and *staying* single. I could fully make this decision based on my own preferences—what I thought was best for Jonathan and for my career. I wouldn't have to worry about a spouse finding employment in a new locale.

* * *

After a year of clinical training, I had learned a lot about medicine and caring for patients, but I was also learning about what doctors do. These were subtle rules—nothing written down or explicitly told to students—learned through observation on the wards. These rules were not necessarily right or wrong, but in clinical rotation after clinical rotation, they were consistent:

- Doctors take the stairs, not the elevator.
- Doctors walk briskly.
- Doctors tuck in their scrubs.
- Doctors are confident and don't express doubt and if there is uncertainty, doctors are definitive in discussing possibilities.
- Doctors are professional.
- Doctors don't get sick (well, they do, but they don't call in sick).
- Doctors don't require much sleep.
- Doctors don't cry in front of patients (if they cry at all).
- Doctors—not nurses, social workers, or aides—deliver bad news.

At 5 a.m. every day, I arrived at the hospital to do my usual "pre-rounding." I checked lab and imaging results and saw how patients were doing before meeting with the attending to do formal rounds. One day, I saw that a patient had unfortunate results. The X-ray and CT scan revealed a large mass in his chest cavity. There also appeared to be metastases. The image on the computer screen revealed much about why the patient had been weak, coughing up blood, losing weight, experiencing shortness of breath, and suffering chest pain. When the attending, Dr. Lee, arrived on the unit, I shared the results of the imaging.

"Dr. Lee, there's bad news about Mr. Brown, the fifty-four-year-old gentleman who presented to the emergency room yesterday with shortness of breath and chest pain. He is in room D4, bed 2, and his CT scan results are back."

Dr. Lee was an Asian male who, although short in stature, was intimidating in terms of knowledge and bedside manner. He wore small, thin-rimmed glasses. He exemplified what being a doctor meant, and I imagined that even without his long, white coat, he would still look like a physician.

"So what are you going to tell him?" he asked me.

I hesitated. I wasn't quite sure if I had heard the question correctly. Was this a rhetorical, "Oh, what would you tell the patient if you were his doctor?" . . . or an" Oh, what are you thinking in terms of diagnosis, treatment, and prognosis?" What was he really asking?

"Well, I would tell him that he has lung cancer and that we would need additional lab work and studies. Likely a biopsy. He will need to be referred to heme-onc—"

He interrupted me while he simultaneously looked at the computer screen and scrolled through the images of the patient's CT scan.

"Is that how you are going to tell him he has cancer? Cancer with metastases? Terminal cancer?"

Again, I didn't know whether he was getting at how I would deliver bad news if I were the attending.

"Well, if I were the attending," I acknowledged, deferring to him, "I'd make sure he has a support person in the room, and if he doesn't, I'd ask him if he would like that. Then I'd tell him directly. I'd try not to give him too much information." I tried to sound matter-of-fact. I was thinking back to all the times I'd observed attendings giving bad news while I, as the medical student, stood alongside, not uttering a word. Delivering bad news wasn't my role as a medical student.

"This morning, you are going to tell the patient he has lung cancer."

"Me?" I looked at him as if he was asking me to climb Mt. Kilimanjaro.

"Yes, you, Melanie. You have spent significant time with this patient since yesterday morning. Actually, more time than I have been able to. If the doctor doesn't deliver difficult news, who does?"

I knew he was right, but I was expecting to do this much later in my career, perhaps as a resident. Was it fair to the patient to hear this devastating news from a medical student? But Dr. Lee was right. I had spent more time with the patient than he had; the news might be more awkward coming from him. Dr. Lee would not ask me to do this if he didn't feel I was mature and capable enough to do it. Part of my sub-internship was handling more responsibility. In any event, I would have to start doing this difficult job eventually.

"I'll give you a few minutes to collect your thoughts. Let's meet outside of his room at 9:15."

How was I to spend the next few minutes? Should I practice my wording? Should I review the recent literature and data about prognosis? No, not that; without a biopsy I wouldn't know what to tell him, though I knew from the imaging that it didn't look good. What if he asked a question I couldn't answer? Was Dr. Lee even going to be in the room? My heart raced. How was Mr. Brown going to respond? Would he yell? Would he cry? Would he say I gave him inaccurate information?

I decided to pray.

I took a deep breath and asked God to give me the strength to share this information with the patient. I asked God to be with Mr. Brown while he received it. I prayed in the bathroom until 9:13. I asked God to give me the words and to equip me to handle Mr. Brown's reaction appropriately.

I walked towards room D4, bed 2, knowing the patient's life would never be the same after I conveyed the news. He didn't just have pneumonia or tuberculosis. It was cancer.

Dr. Lee approached the room at the same time I arrived. He nodded to me, as if to ask silently if I was ready. I nodded back. My body language would be important, so instead of hugging my clipboard to my chest as I was tempted to do, I held it by my side. I had silenced my pager so there wouldn't be any distractions. I reached to close the door behind me, but I was relieved to see that Dr. Lee was following me in. He stood behind me and to the side, at the five o'clock position, very much the place I would normally have taken in this scenario. It was up to me.

Mr. Brown was eating breakfast. He didn't seem very ill. He didn't look as though he could run a marathon, but he didn't appear weak or frail, either. He acknowledged our presence and placed his fork on his plate.

"Hello, doctors." He coughed after speaking.

"Good morning, Mr. Brown," I said, knowing it wouldn't be a good morning, a good day, a good evening, or a good week or month for Mr. Brown.

"Tony, please," he said. "Please, call me Tony"

"Tony, we have the results of your CT scan."

"Okay. Is everything all right? This cough has been nagging me."

"I have some news to share with you. Would you like someone to be here with you?"

Anxiety spread across his face. "No, there's no one here. Whatever you have to say, I'll hear it."

"Okay." I paused. "It appears that you have cancer—lung cancer."

Silence.

More silence.

"Are you sure?" he said finally. "I thought maybe it was pneumonia. I'm too young to have cancer, right?"

What to do? Should I rattle off statistics about lung cancer in his age group? Should I give him data on smokers versus nonsmokers?

"Yes, both your chest X-ray and CT scan showed a large mass and what appears to be metastases; that is, the cancer has spread. I'm so sorry"

I wanted to ask him if he had questions, so there would be something to fill the silence, but I was afraid he would ask a question to which I had no answer. The silence became excruciatingly uncomfortable.

"So, what to do now?" he finally asked.

I looked towards Dr. Lee, who didn't chime in. This was all on me.

"We need to obtain more laboratory work. We will need a biopsy to get more information on the type of lung cancer it is. From there, we can talk about the most appropriate treatment, such as surgery, radiation, or chemotherapy."

"Will I need all of that?"

"We won't know until we get a little more information."

I knew that only so much was going to sink in. I had learned this from previously observing doctors deliver bad news. More questions tended to come up later.

"Is there anyone you'd like me to call?" I asked. "Please let me know if I can help you with telling any loved ones."

He shook his head no and looked out the window. Our visit, for now, was done.

* * *

26

In all the years of Jonathan's life, I had never really sat down with him and discussed his father's absence. For the short term, the explanation of different families are different had sufficed. Jonathan was aware that some families only had a mommy, some only had a daddy, some had a mommy and daddy who lived apart from each other, and some had loving grandparents but no mommy or daddy. I often pointed out these differences, but I was unable to talk with Jonathan about our specific situation.

I finally decided that if I had almost graduated from medical school and could tell a patient he had terminal cancer, I had to be mature enough to handle this delicate, difficult conversation with Jonathan. Darryl's absence was our "elephant in the room," a topic that was never fully addressed but was painfully apparent at birthday parties, at Christmas time, and on Father's Day. It was also evident at Jonathan's soccer games, basketball games, and swimming practices.

I couldn't believe how anxious I was about bringing up the subject. In the past, I'd only superficially mentioned the topic as it came up on Father's Day or father/child events at his school, but I had to plunge in … go deeper. I found I couldn't do it face-to-face, so one day I brought it up while driving, when Jonathan was in the back seat of the car. This was one of the times I was happy that he preferred to sit in the back while being chauffeured around. I didn't want to see him cry. I didn't want him to be sad about a situation I could not control. But I had my own personal concerns. Darryl's ongoing absence brought up many issues for me, too. I didn't want to really accept that throughout all these years, I had never been able to remarry and provide Jonathan a father. And I didn't know how to explain why his biological father didn't accept that role. How much to tell an eight-year-old boy?

"Jonathan, do you ever think about your dad?"

He didn't hesitate. In true eight-year-old fashion, he asked several questions in a row: "Do you have pictures of him? Does he look like me? Where does he live? What is his name?"

"His name is Darryl, and he lives in Mississippi." I didn't finish the full sentence in my mind, the sentence that ended in, "I think." It had been so long that I couldn't say for sure that he still lived there.

"Where is Mississippi? Can we drive there?"

I took a deep breath. Is he going to want to meet him now? What had I started? I wasn't ready for all of this.

"It's more like a plane ride than a drive, Jonathan."

"Oh ... can he come *here*?"

The conversation was getting more challenging. I looked up to the roof of the car and sighed a little, trying to hide my building frustration.

"Well, sometimes things don't work out between grown-ups. When you were little, I didn't know whether he could be a good daddy for you." I wondered if I should have said that, but I continued, "I can show you pictures, and I can answer your questions."

He didn't say anything, and so I went on.

"There are men in your life who do 'daddy things' with you, right? Who are they?"

"Mark, Ian ..."

I mentioned some more men—my male classmates, my mentors, our pastor.

"Oh yeah."

"Not every family has a daddy," I said.

"And not every family has a mommy," he responded.

I didn't tell him what a rare occurrence that is and how most single parents are women.

"Yes, that's true."

We arrived at our destination. He got out of the back seat, and I gave him a hug. I had finally initiated the conversation I had been dreading for years. I was sure there would be more conversations in the future, but at least I had started.

* * *

Fall of 2002 was the beginning of interview season for residencies. I interviewed at several different programs in California, Massachusetts, Missouri, and Arizona. I didn't have any real strategy other than choosing programs that had strong OB/GYN residencies and a few where I had family or friends nearby. My experience at Stanford made me a bit cocky about building a support system wherever I went. If I had managed it so well there, why couldn't I recreate it *anywhere?*

. I did my best to prepare for interviews, staging mock interviews with friends and attendings, reading books on common residency interview questions, and trying to come up with a strategy. Some students advocated interviewing first for the programs that one was least interested in so as to get the practice. Others believed in interviewing at the top places first since you would be fresh and enthusiastic, then burnt-out and less animated by the ninth or tenth interview. Burnout was a real danger. All the time, money, and resources involved in interviewing were nothing to take lightly. It was a significant investment to purchase a nice suit, fly across the country (at times with little notice), stay in a hotel, and arrange transportation.

My first interviews were at Harvard. Fortunately, I would be able to interview at two of the Harvard-affiliated OB/GYN residency programs on the same trip to Boston. Ian would take care of Jonathan at home. These interviews would be the most challenging, in part because of the programs' prestige, and also because of the weather. It was snowing in Boston. The good news was that, thanks to Weight Watchers, I was about thirty pounds lighter. Although the suit I had worn as a college student interviewing for medical school was too small, I had more confidence now. I was interviewing as a Stanford medical student for a Harvard residency program. I was proud of my accomplishments.

Fortunately, I had no hotel bills. Dr. Allison, with whom I had worked during my maternal-fetal medicine (high-risk obstetrics) rotation, offered to let me stay at her home, which was only ten minutes away from the Harvard-affiliated hospitals. It was most unusual for an attending to host a medical student, but she had taken a liking to me, and, most importantly, she was also a parent. She knew how difficult balancing family and academics could be. She would be out of town for the week at a convention, but she left a key in a hidden spot. I arrived at 10 p.m. after a flight delay and headed directly upstairs to the bedroom.

I couldn't sleep. I couldn't shut my mind down. I debated on whether to take a Benadryl, but I was anxious about a hangover effect. I didn't want to be drowsy at my interview. And then went the internal debate—"drowsy versus bags under the eyes." It was 11:35 p.m., then 12:10 a.m. I had to get up in five hours to be at the hospital at 7 a.m. I *had* to get some sleep. Reluctantly, I took a Benadryl. I woke up to the buzzing of an alarm clock, but the clock had been buzzing for forty-five minutes! I'd slept through the alarm, something that had never happened before. Never! I called a taxi. I almost said I needed it stat. There wasn't time to shower. I tried to put on my pantyhose while on the phone with the cab company. They were too tight. I dug my nail in, and they tore. I shouted an expletive and threw the hose away. I put on my bra, my shirt, and my suit. I looked at myself in the mirror. I was a horrible combination of drowsy *with* bags under eyes. I splashed my face with cold water, grabbed a damp washcloth to take with me, and smoothed my hair back into a tight bun. I would put on earrings and make-up in the cab. I took my briefcase and made it downstairs just as the taxi was pulling up.

My adrenaline competed with my tears. I couldn't let myself cry—not one tear.

"I'll give you a ten-dollar tip if you can get me to the Brigham as soon as possible, please."

The taxicab driver nodded and did his best given the snow and traffic. I prayed and prayed. "Lord, please help me, please. I've travelled so far for this. This can't be happening!" I tried to put on my pearl earrings, but I lost a backing on the floor. It was too tiny to find. Self-doubt overcame me. Maybe I was not meant to do this. What was I thinking? I rocked back and forth in the back seat. No pantyhose, no earrings, no class. I smeared some deodorant under my arms, trying to avoid getting any on my suit. Sweat formed on my forehead, on my neck, and across my chest. There wouldn't be time to stop at the bathroom. I blotted my face and neck with the washcloth.

The taxi got me to the hospital at 7:18 a.m. Too late! I gave the cabbie a twenty and yelled, "Thanks" as I slammed the door. I raced up to the main entrance and looked at the interview itinerary. My interview was on the fourth floor. Stairs or elevator? What if I missed my interview while I was in the elevator? But the stairs would leave me out of breath. Since I was wearing heels, I opted for the elevator.

I entered a waiting area where the receptionist greeted me. "Yes, Dr. Watkins," she said. "You arrived just in time. Take a deep breath. You're just fine." I appreciated her reassurance. She handed me a name badge and directed me to a large conference room. Approximately fifteen other people in standard blue or black suits sat around a large table, eating pastries and drinking coffee and juice. Many of them looked my way as I walked in. I slid right into a seat. Two minutes later, the residency director, who was familiar to me from the previous summer, entered the room.

"Welcome to Brigham and Women's Hospital."

Praise God. I had made it. I wasn't too late. It was going to be all right. Next time, I would set three alarms. Next time, I'd wear clip-on earrings. Next time, I'd bring an extra pair of pantyhose. But for now, I would set those thoughts aside and do the best I could on this interview and leave the rest to God.

* * *

When I finally wrapped up the interviews, and again, I realized how much of my life had been spent doing "school, study, sleep, see Jon" repeat. It was nice to have a bit of a break as clinical rotations and interviews were completed. Jonathan was involved in basketball through the local YMCA, and I took him and his friend to their game. They looked so happy and carefree as they dribbled the ball back and forth across the court. They were having fun. Jonathan had no idea how much anxiety I had felt in putting together the rank list that I submitted the previous day. I prayed to God I was making the right decision, and yet I felt so far from God. I hadn't spent much time seeking Him or praying to Him unless I needed guidance or wanted a particular outcome. I hadn't given much thanks for all that had occurred, but I imagined God must be somewhat understanding of this. He did make me human, right? So despite feeling I was continually asking Him to do something for me without expressing gratitude, I apologized and prayed for guidance. I needed Him to show me the way.

For the OB/GYN residency programs, I had decided to rank UCSF first and the Brigham Hospital in Boston second. I wondered why I had done this. Why had I chosen hospitals approximately three thousand miles apart? I had made connections in Boston while I completed my sub-internship in maternal-fetal medicine there in the summer, and people there seemed to think I could create a support system in that location. However, the weather was intimidating. I'd had only a small taste of it in March, but I realized how much snow can slow you down.

At UCSF, I'd be only forty-five minutes north of Palo Alto, and some of my classmates were also hoping to match there. The residents had seemed genuine, down-to-earth, and supportive. But then I had second thoughts and doubted my decision. That program was for those interested in academics. Could I do academics? Did I potentially want even more training after residency, such as a fellowship in high-risk obstetrics, infertility, or women's cancers? Did I want to publish journal articles and teach residents? I wasn't quite sure, but I did know I wanted to have a good education and be among the best in the field.

Should I have tried to stay at Stanford? I had support there, but faculty and friends advised me to diversify my training and go elsewhere for residency. I had thought of Santa Clara Valley Medical Center, where I had enjoyed doing most of my rotations. There, I'd be highly involved and likely doing more procedures than at an academic center, but I might not have as much access to faculty who wrote textbooks and published the latest articles.

I was torn. What was best for my career, and what was best for Jonathan? What if I had made the wrong decision? Once a student is matched, there is no turning back. One can't start an internship and then in a few months say, "Oh, I think I'd rather train at another hospital." That would leave the program without an intern, which would mean more work for the other residents to cover, residents who already worked eighty hours a week. Secondly, it would mean trying to find a program elsewhere, many of which would have no empty slots. For all intents and purposes, this was a permanent decision, much like getting a tattoo or a vasectomy.

I couldn't sleep for weeks before match day. I'd had difficulty sleeping ever since the Boston interviews in March. Before that, I had always been able fall asleep without difficulty, perhaps because I was chronically sleep-deprived. Part of my anxiety was facing the realization that I could not change the rank order list. It was out of my hands at this point. But I didn't even know if I *wanted* to change the rank order list.

The day arrived in March, 2003. Match day. We gathered in a large lobby at the medical school, and the dean discussed the importance of the day. But we already knew how it important it was. The speech wasn't really necessary, and I don't think many of us really heard what he said. Family and friends filled the entire lobby. We all stood, almost shoulder-to-shoulder. We would soon learn our fates for the next one to eight years. A reporter from the Stanford newspaper asked if he could write about my thoughts on match day. I accepted his offer, despite feeling light-headed and giddy. My pulse, and that of eighty of my classmates, was palpable without the touch of two fingers on the wrist or a stethoscope on the chest. Medical students across the country were about to learn their fates.

Khadijah, a classmate a few years behind me, was by my side. She was another African-American student who had expressed some interest in pursuing a career in OB/GYN. I liked the thought of mentoring her. Ob/GYN was not one of the specialties on that "road" to happiness. It was becoming a less popular choice due to the work hours, the long nights on call, the rising malpractice insurance premiums, and concerns about lawsuits. However, I enjoyed it. I liked witnessing birth and talking with women about their concerns. I enjoyed the intimacy of it all. I liked providing education and support. The pace, while anxiety-provoking at times, was also a wild adrenaline rush, and I liked the idea of being the doctor to come in and save the day—to stop the bleeding, to get the baby out, to stop the pain.

Our envelopes in hand, it was now time to learn our fates. Three hours away in Boston, New York, and other East Coast cities, medical students were also opening envelopes. Khadijah was close, and I almost wanted her to open the envelope, but I didn't want to show her my anxiety. I opened the envelope:

University of California, San Francisco: Obstetrics and Gynecology

Khadijah screamed. She wrapped her arm around me, and the reporter took a picture. I was in shock. I got my first choice! But I nevertheless felt a sense of panic. I was going to become an OB/GYN. I was going to train at a top program on the West Coast. I was going be a single mom working eighty hours a week in San Francisco, where I had no support system in place, where there were likely more pet owners than parents. Where would Jon go to school?

My thoughts raced. I was still panicking. I just wanted to leave the room. All of the medical students were crying, laughing, smiling, and screaming. Many Stanford students do get their first, second, or third choices. But I still wondered whether this was really the best choice for me. I'd never had a panic attack, but this came close. I feigned a smile to my classmates and said my congratulations. All I wanted was to pick Jonathan up from school, take him home, and squeeze him tightly. I prayed that I had made the right decision for us.

* * *

A few weeks later, I had finally let the news sink in. My friends and attendings reassured me that my anxiety was normal. I would be starting residency in July. As God had done in the past, He continued to provide me with the resources Jonathan and I needed. Through a mutual friend, I met Linda, another single mother with a child close to Jonathan's age. She was an orthopedics resident in her third year of training at USCF. Linda was a strong, assertive physician in her mid-thirties who was originally from San Francisco. We decided to share a home and a nanny for our children, and I moved into the house she was renting. The OB/GYN residents were warm and welcoming. There were other black female residents with whom I connected. Although there were not any other single parents in the obstetrics and gynecology residency program, other residents had children before and during residency.

Mom traveled from Reno to my graduation from Stanford. We invited my friends, classmates, and mentors to a breakfast party at my apartment that morning. As I watched my mother make quiche and prepare for the guests, I thought about her in a different way. She had never been the mother I really wanted. She wasn't the mother who called often to check in, who gave lots of hugs, who sent special gifts, or who would listen to me cry about a setback at school, but she was the mother I needed. She did help me with Jonathan in difficult times, and she was trying to be a better mom. Even what I perceived as her lack of support made me stronger and more resilient. Because I couldn't solely depend on her, I'd frequently been forced to find other ways to manage my life. I also realized that I hadn't been the easiest daughter, and I had placed some unanticipated challenges in her life, such as making her a grandmother at forty-six. Only now, with the eyes of an adult and a parent, could I see my mother as a human being with her own life, dreams, and goals. She was trying to do what she could to help in the only way she knew how.

That morning, I was surrounded by family and friends who knew how special this day was for both Jonathan and me. I thought about all the sacrifices and disappointments. I thought about the support and the joy. I had spent four years in college and five years at Stanford. Nine years down, and four to go. I would graduate with the title of Dr. Watkins, a role that would take me several years to grow into.

There wouldn't be much time between graduation and starting internship. We would have to move to San Francisco just a few days after graduation. At the ceremony, Jonathan was unaware that I was looking at him. I thought about him as a baby and remembered those days when we took the bus while loaded down with backpack, baby bag, and stroller. I thought about the days I brought him to school with me when there weren't any childcare options. I thought about him playing with my organic chemistry set or drawing in my anatomy textbook. I thought about being up all night with him when he was ill. I thought about reading him bedtime stories and how he had memorized them and "read" them back to me. At times, he had read to me until I fell asleep because I was too tired to stay awake.

At graduation, he wore a suit and clip-on tie. He laughed with adults and kids while I waited with classmates for the processional. He had such pride and happiness, as if it were his graduation, too. Indeed, Jonathan was the same age as my education. I had been in school his entire life. When my name was called to receive my diploma, Jonathan joined me on the stage. The audience applauded and cheered. This was the beginning of a better life for us. We had made it through first steps, first year of medical school, first grade. No doubt we'd make it through internship, elementary school, and residency, too. We were growing up together.

* * *

Afterword

My internship in OB/GYN began at UCSF in the summer of 2003. While there, I had the opportunity to deliver hundreds of babies. It was a blessing to be in the delivery room and witness birth—to be the first person to place my hands on a new life. It was also thrilling to learn the steps of doing a hysterectomy or resolving a woman's discomfort or heavy bleeding by providing medication or doing surgical procedures. But I realized that one of the main reasons I wanted to be an obstetrician/gynecologist was because I enjoyed talking with patients, particularly young patients, not only about their reproductive health, but also about their living situations, their backgrounds, and their support systems. I enjoyed the intimacy of hearing their stories, their stressors, and their concerns, but the fast pace of being an obstetrician/gynecologist didn't allow me the opportunity to connect with patients as much as I would have liked. In addition, I gained back the weight I'd lost during my last months of medical school. As a resident, it was not uncommon to work long hours, and overnight call was expected as part of the training. Exhaustion was competing with the exhilaration of the deliveries and procedures. After sixteen months of training, I decided to take a leave of absence for a month. During this time, I was seeking guidance and support from colleagues and mentors. I learned more about the field of psychiatry—one in which I could have more time to spend with patients and to have a lifestyle that would allow me to spend more time with Jonathan. After this time of contemplation and introspection, I decided to pursue a position as a resident in psychiatry.

My training in psychiatry began in January 2005. Psychiatry did seem a better fit for me, and I cherished the amount of time I could spend getting to know my patients while learning all aspects of their care. I learned a lot about myself as well in the process. Psychiatry not only allowed me to be more involved with Jonathan, but I was able to work on my weight loss goals. Fortunately, I was able to return to Weight Watchers and lost ninety pounds in my first year of psychiatry training. After completing that goal, I felt I could do anything, and I decided to train for a marathon. Completing my first marathon in 2007 was a metaphor for my life. With marathon training, there is time for preparation and practice, a time to give it your all on the 26.2 mile stretch, a time to celebrate at the finish line with family and friends, and then a time to reflect on all of it in the days following. Indeed, this memoir is itself a reflection on how far I've come in the "marathon" of my medical training and mothering.

Today, I spend time practicing medicine at a county hospital and in a small private practice. I do enjoy public speaking and cherish the opportunity to share my story at high schools, community organizations, and churches. It is interesting to speak at high schools and talk with students who are sixteen, the same age as Jonathan is now and the same age I was when I became pregnant. I know all too well many of the challenges they face. We, as a society, need to encourage young people to make good choices and to understand that all choices have consequences. I tell teenagers that I believe it is better to wait until there is a good foundation in place before starting a family. It is also good to be accountable to oneself and one's community. It is important to have faith in something bigger than oneself. My personal faith is in God, who gave me the strength and determination to make it through some very trying times. As has been said by others, He placed the right people in my life at the times I needed them the most.

Young people need the support of adults in helping them to make good decisions and provide guidance. I am often asked, "How did you beat the odds?" I did so because people believed in me, both at the times when I felt confident that I could do it, and also when I doubted my abilities. Their consistent belief in me made the difference. None of what I achieved would have been possible without significant emotional, spiritual, logistical, and financial support from friends, mentors, colleagues, and yes, even strangers, who generously donated funds for the many scholarships and grants

I received as a college and medical student. To all of them, the best gift I can give is to provide that support and encourage others to do the same for young people striving to achieve their dreams. To them, I say, "Thank you for giving me the opportunity to 'pay it forward.'"

* * *

Acknowledgements

"Trust in the Lord with all your heart and lean not on your own understanding. In all your ways acknowledge Him and He shall direct your path." Proverbs 3:5-6

Mentors and Doctors: Thank you for believing that I could achieve my dreams. Alice (Arndt) Heiman, Barbara King, Andre Thorn, Anne Firth Murray, Dr. Thornton, Dr. Gubanich, Dr. Mead, Dr. LeBaron, Dr. Winkleby and her husband Dr. Mike, Dr. Litwin-Sanguinetti, Dr. Mason, Dr. Matthews, Dr. Graves, Dr. LeMay, Dr. Tam Chang, Dr. Osias, Dr. Price, Dr. Vincent, Pastor and Mrs. Taylor, Pastor and Mrs. Harrison, Jack Canfield and Mark Victor Hansen from the Chicken Soup Series.

Family and friends: Thank you for your love and support. My mother Dorothy Walton, my sister Tonya Ware, the Watkins brothers, Elaine and my nieces and nephews, Aunt Bertha Salter, Arthur and Linda White, Mark and Ian a.k.a. "the mannies". The Escondido Village community at Stanford University. The Nevada Women's Fund, The USA Today All-USA Academic Team Selection Committee, and Lifetime Television. Staff and students at the University of Nevada Reno, Stanford University and the University of California, San Francisco. And to all of my good friends throughout the years—thank you for being there for Jonathan and me.

* * *